DENY YOUR INSTINCTS TO SURVIVE

A Healthy Weightloss Guide with a Twist

By your Phat Phriend Charlie Goodnight

If one more person says, "If you want to lose weight, all you have to do is diet & exercise," I'm going to pie them in the face. Dang I love pie. But I also love being healthy. Can we have both? Can we have a lifestyle where we can enjoy our food and be healthy at the same time? I'm so excited to share with you that the answer is YES! This book has the juicy secrets that will allow you to be satisfied with your food and yourself at the same exact time.

Since the creation of mankind, our bodies were created to store extra calories. This survival instinct is what kept humans alive through famine, plagues, droughts, and long winters. One look in the mirror shows me that my ancestors survived some very long winters. Our instincts tell us to eat what tastes good, and to eat as much of it as possible. To reach your health goals, you will have to:

Deny Your Instincts to Survive.

Join me on a journey of health. Join me in between diets. Join me in the deep places of your soul that require confidence so that you can meet the health goals you have always wanted, yet never attained. We will laugh together, we might cry too. One thing is for certain; you will end this book mentally stronger on your health journey.

How to read this book:

Upside down. Read it alone, or read it with an accountability group. Read it with a good cup of coffee and a friend. Read it all in one sitting or read one chapter a week. Read it in the rain or on a treadmill. Put it on the shelf, then get it back down and read it again. Read it until you don't need it. Welcome friends, to the first day of the rest of your life.

Table of Contents

INTRODUCTION:

THE JUICY SECRET

This book will change your life. It's like when you find out the person you love is cheating on you, or that you have a long lost sibling somewhere, or that a cell phone can have 10 times more bacteria than a toilet seat... Once you know, you can never un-know.

So raise a toast, here's to the rest of your changed life: a thriving life.

Ever spend all day loathing what you see in the mirror, or how you feel in your pants? Yet somehow we desperately long for a pint of ice-cream at the end of the day? OK, lets be honest, a gallon of ice-cream? How often do we come up with a million excuses not to exercise? But when you actually do exercise you feel amazing! WHAT THE HECK IS GOING ON! Why do we do the things we hate, and hate the things we do?

Our feelings and desires war against our souls that truly longing for a healthy body. We are at constant war in our minds over what we "should" do vs. what we "feel" like doing. If you are anything like me, I was trapped here for a very long time: wanting to be healthy and not being able to do so. I've started thousands of perfectly healthy days. But then I would get out of bed and well, you know, life happens. Can you relate? So let's get unstuck together.

This isn't a book for the person who eats whatever they want and stays thin. I hate that person (but really I love you and I really want to be you). This is for the person who just looks at cake and gains ten pounds. Those are my people. This isn't for the person who has devoted their life to fitness and spends six hours a day at the gym and makes millions. You stink. Literally. This is for the person who is too embarrassed to go to the gym because it's covered in mirrors. This is a book for the person who feels like they can't even get one aspect of their life right. You are in good company.

Together, we will implement small achievable changes that will literally save our lives. The rest of this book is about day-to-day choices that will help you achieve the health goals you are longing for. This playbook will create the bridge from feeling stuck to taking back control of your health.

Let's do this.

CHAPTER ONE

CELEBRATE

Stop what you are doing, take a second, and celebrate. Unless you are reading this book; don't stop doing that. Well clearly you are reading this book. So just ignore the stop part. Keep reading. Celebrate that you— right this very second— are taking a step in the right direction on your health journey. Sure, if you're like me, you still have a long way to go. Don't miss the battle victories! Go ahead. Get jiggy with it. Dance it out. High five yourself. Work it. Twerk it. Bump it. Drop it like its hot. Great job.

Very few people are motivated by pessimistic criticism. But isn't that exactly how we talk to ourselves regarding our bodies? Quit it. Instead, celebrate.

For example, I was going through a Starbucks drive-through to order a pumpkin spice latte. I enjoy one each year. As I ordered in sheer jubilation, I was doing a little dance in my car. Picture Shakira meets Steve Urkel. Suddenly the barista's voice came through the speaker in a roar of laughter. I froze and said, "You can see me can't you."

"Yes my dear. Yes, I can."

So we laughed together. Go ahead. Dance it out. You know you want to. Shimmy those shoulders.

Today, you might not be able to cut out all your unhealthy carbs. You might not be able to exercise for an hour. However, you are reading this book. You are taking care of yourself by strengthening your mind. Isn't that where the battle lies anyway? Celebrate that you have a body to take care of. Celebrate all the cool things your body does: your senses, your interesting thoughts, your instinctive responses to danger, your curiosities, your aching desire to grow, your ability to run a 4 minute mile when you see a giant spider even though you haven't run a day in your life...

Celebrate reading this book, and every single victory of progress you make along this lifelong journey of health. I have a feeling this is the beginning of a lot of celebrating.

Group Discussion Questions:

1. What holds you back from celebrating your progress?
2. Have you been excited about your health journey in the past? What happened?
3. How have failures in the past prevented you from moving forward in your health journey?
4. How will you celebrate moving forward?
5. Why should you celebrate?

CHAPTER TWO

CELEBRATE WITH FOOD

My favorite lesson of all: **celebrate with food.**

Now, I'm not talking about "going out for ice cream because it's Tuesday, and Tuesdays aren't Mondays, so we should celebrate with food" kind of celebrating. I'm talking about treating yourself to a tasty healthy meal, like your favorite salad or blackened salmon with a side of roasted veggies. The main gist of this book, the crux that will help you finally and once and for all kick those unhealthy habits, is to *change your mindset.*

Right now, if you are like me, celebrating usually includes the sweetest, saltiest, fattiest foods we can imagine. That's not celebrating. That's punishment. Sure, for a few divine seconds your taste buds are totally titillated. But then you stop tasting. You keep eating. You look around to see if anyone has noticed the enormous portions on your plate. You get seconds and eat in a different room so people don't know its your second plate. Maybe thirds. Then you walk by the buffet table and just pick up anything and put it in your mouth with your back turned so people don't necessarily know you are eating. Guilt. Shame. Regret. Self-Loathing. Punishment. Quit it.

Celebrate with food instead.

One of the Merriam-Webster definitions of celebrate is: "to honor (an occasion, such as a holiday) especially by solemn ceremonies or by refraining from ordinary business." Let's change it up a bit:

> **Celebrate: To honor one's self by eating life-giving food and by refraining from eating the ordinary food that is destroying one's body.**

Maybe the words "healthy food" make you gag. You're in good company. You are NOT destined to a life of obesity and food addiction. But you do have to participate. The good news is, you have already begun. You are taking steps to change your mind, which will change your actions. Right thinking leads to right behavior.

So here are some ways you can celebrate with food:

Try a new recipe! Go to your favorite restaurant that has your very favorite healthy meal. Don't have one? Try a tour of restaurants that offer salads until you find one! Sure, some salads are over one thousand calories. Let's just start putting salads in your diet. Then we can work on what kinds of salads are healthier.

Group Discussion Questions:

1. How has food been part of your life celebrations?
2. How can you enjoy traditional celebrations without destroying your body with unhealthy food?
3. How will you celebrate with food?
4. Do you have any healthy recipes you can share with the group?

5. What restaurant has your favorite salad? Better yet, make a date with your group to start your epic salad tour. Come up with a cute group name and make every waiter or waitress uncomfortable by laughing at it when you tell them what you call yourselves. High five!

CHAPTER THREE

DON'T DIET OR EXERCISE

Wouldn't we all love to have a rock star body? Wouldn't it be nice to get a perfect bill of health at every doctor visit? Of course we all desire to be healthy. So why, then, are over 160 million Americans overweight? Turning desire into reality is maybe the greatest psychological struggle of modern America: the American Dream, if you will. I'll tell you the very best place to start.

Don't diet or exercise.

Instead, take care of your mental and emotional health. I promise the diet and exercise will come a lot easier when you are in a good place mentally and emotionally.

I had had one of those mornings. My kids woke up too early and it was nonstop "Mom" this and "Mom" that. Potty training, nursing a baby, homeschooling, getting our immigration visa's denied. My life was full of stress. I was drained, empty, exhausted. I wanted to bury myself in the bottom of an ice-cream container... at nine in the morning. The thought of going out and exercising felt like a disappointing chore. Quite like my six year old felt when, Lord forbid, I asked her to pick up her shoes. Luckily I was able to escape the blissful chaos of home and get to a local café. As I sat, listening to smooth jazz, chugging coffee, and reading a borderline trashy vampire romance novel, I felt myself take a deep breath. Suddenly, the prospect of ordering healthy food and getting some exercise sounded quite refreshing!

Let's be honest, if you're reading this book, you probably have more than ten pounds to lose. I've been there: four times. I had to commit years to losing weight in order to achieve my "goal weight." There were bad weeks. But I still did it: four times. I've also been able to keep the weight off since the last time I lost 50 pounds. I don't have to diet anymore because my lifestyle is one where I enjoy food, stay healthy, and eat cake. It is possible. I dare you to believe me.

You can too. The point is, don't give up because you've had a bad streak. Remember, this is a long-term goal. This is a life change. Unless you are a fitness/wellness professional, you're probably going to have a bad streak at some point. Don't give up because of that. Acknowledge it, brainstorm ways to do better in the same circumstances, and move on.

Everyone knows a healthy diet and exercise are amazing ways to take care of your body and mind. In fact, they have a direct impact on the success of your emotional and psychological health! But sometimes you have to put the chicken before the egg. Take care of your psychological health, manage your stress, read a good book or take a nap. Fill up your soul so your soul can meet your body. Then, pick yourself up and handle it. Own it. Wreck it. Be the better version of yourself that you've always known you could be.

Group Discussion Questions:

1. What are the biggest emotional obstacles to taking steps toward your health?
2. What lies do you believe that are holding you back?

3. What factors lead to your "bad weeks?" How can you fight them next time?
4. What fills your emotional tank? How can you include more of this in your life?
5. What healthy stress management technique work for you?

CHAPTER FOUR

UNDERSTANDING INSTINCTS

For the first time in the history of America, it is harder to starve than it is to be obese. Since creation, our bodies have stored any extra calories as fat because a time would be coming when you might not eat. It was the only way the human species survived for thousands of years. Human instinct tells us to eat, eat, eat, then eat more. Our instinct to eat was what kept us alive. Now that same instinct poisons our bodies and souls. We have to deny that innate instinct to constantly eat if we want to survive in this modern world.

Deny your instincts to survive.

One of the main reasons it's impossible for people to lose weight is because it requires changing daily habits... forever. Our conscious and subconscious minds are constantly at war. Consciously we want to be healthy; we want to lose weight. Subconsciously, we eat like we are about to hibernate for nine months. Did you know that even *seeing* food releases the happy hormone, serotonin?

Our subconscious runs the show anytime it can so that our conscious mind can take in new information. Your eating habits live in your subconscious: your instincts if you will. Anytime your conscious mind is working overtime, you will resort to your habitual eating habits.

I gained eight pounds in six weeks one dark winter season. I clearly recall sitting in the doctor's office complaining of chest pain and nausea: I thought I was having a heart attack. I had recently watched an episode of Grey's Anatomy where Chief Miranda Baily almost died of a heart attack. Nausea and chest pain... I was certain that the cream cheese chip dip and cupcakes I had at our family gathering the week before had done me in.

We had only been back in Texas for six weeks to attend my father's funeral. We had flown from Tanzania to Texas with our four children (all under the age of six) to attend the funeral, a wedding, a baby shower, a family reunion, travel to eight different states, get a vasectomy (did you hear me say four children under six?), and God only knows what else we had to do in those few short weeks... As the doctor looked at my EKG results with a concerned look on his face he asks, "Have you been under any stress lately?" Ha!

My EKG was fine. I was having classic anxiety. My mind was so overwhelmed with life that my body was freaking out. My conscious mind was so busy that my lifelong habits of emotional eating were raging. I had been on my health journey for years, but when the burdens of life came crashing down around me, my subconscious mind took over.

It sounds simple enough. Focus on making healthy choices and voila! But if it were that simple, the health industry wouldn't be a billion dollar industry.

So the question is, how do we change our subconscious habits? If we can achieve this, then we won't drown ourselves in calories whenever hard times hit. I'm sure you've heard all the self-help slogans on changing habits:

- It takes seven times to change a habit.
- Repetition and routine.
- Cue, craving, response, reward.
- Change your environment.
- Five steps to changing your habits.
- Etc.

If you Google how to change a habit, you will get over 200,000,000 hits in under half a second. Hear me out, I am NOT discrediting these sources. I'm only illustrating how intensely difficult it is to change unhealthy habits. Some people find the sheer willpower to completely change their lives overnight. Dang, I wish I was one of those people. For others, it takes one baby step at a time. It *is* possible.

Do you know anyone who has:

- Lost weight and kept it off?
- Stopped smoking?
- stopped dating losers and found a good mate?
- Been an alcoholic and stopped drinking?
- Been a drug addict and stopped doing drugs?

You know people first hand who have changed some of the most difficult and destructive habits in the world. You can change some of your habits too. The first step is acknowledging the power of a habit: the subconscious. Now, acknowledge your own unhealthy habits. Take some time to reflect on them. Name them. Talk to a trusted friend or a counselor about them. Instead of pridefully defending them, acknowledge that you want to change. Instead of telling yourself you are not worthy to have healthier habits, believe that your life could be more free if you improved even just one of your unhealthy habits.

Whom the truth sets free, will be free indeed.

Start with the truth. Be honest with yourself. Name the things in your life that are destructive. This isn't just about food. Overeating is a symptom of a greater pain in your life. Name it. Unhealthy boundaries with food probably mean you have some unhealthy boundaries in other areas of your life. What are they? Say them out loud, unless you are reading this in the middle of a coffee shop. Then you will just look cray cray. Write them down instead.

Group Discussion Questions:

1. What are some of your destructive subconscious habits?
2. Where did you learn some of your unhealthy habits?
3. Who shares your unhealthy habits in your daily life?
4. Name a time when you have changed a habit. What were your motivations? Circumstances?
5. What is one habit you want to focus on changing?

CHAPTER FIVE

GET DRUNK (NOT REALLY)

I was sitting at my favorite African coffee shop when I had just finished my fourth cappuccino, or as I like to call it, my cuppa joe. Don't judge me. I'm obsessed with coffee. I drink so many cappuccinos at this place that they don't even ask what I want to drink or if I want a refill. My usual waitress, Jackie, just keeps bringing me coffee until I tell her to stop. The locals don't actually drink coffee so they think I'm a bit of a phenomenon the way I can drink so much coffee and still walk straight when I leave.

Anywho, It was time to go so I went to the counter to pay my bill. This restaurant is in a part of the world where you don't leave your purse at the table while you go to the restroom. You paint a picture of yourself on the hubcaps of your car so they don't get stolen. You don't wear fancy jewelry in public. You tie your car keys to a rope around your waist. You get the point. On this particular day, I had a wallet stacked with cash because it was payday for the nanny and everyone gets paid in cash here.

As I turned to leave, I absentmindedly left my wallet on the counter. The next thing I hear is "Muzungu!" That is a slang word for foreigner. "You left your money. The coffee made you drunk." Hey thanks bud. I then went and ran 15 miles that day on caffeine alone. Just kidding.

Get drunk my friends. Get drunk on water!!!! Look, alcohol has an unbelievable amount of calories and sugars that really do destroy your efforts to eat healthy and exercise. However, water is miraculous. It increases your metabolism, helps your body process out all the junk inside, and tells your stomach you are not ravenously hungry for a country style buffet.

I used to live in Uganda where we had to take five-gallon jugs to the nearby stream to get water. We then had to boil the water and strain it to get out any sediment. It took hours to cool. It was only served at room temperature. This is how millions of people in the world live today. Chances are, none of you who are reading this book have had to work that hard for safe drinking water. So you probably take it for granted. Water can feel mundane in the western world. The truth is, water, which is most of the time free, is one of the most life sustaining substances in the world! I always laugh out loud when I see the brand Smart Water. It's really smart to buy something I can get for free. Lolz.

I had a best friend in high school named Drue. Her mom used to always say, "You should eat your calories, don't drink them." So I started drinking diet sodas. Then I realized my sugar cravings went through the roof. My tastebuds were telling my brain that I needed more sugar. I actually lost weight when I stopped drinking diet sodas and started drinking water.

Water can help prevent you from overeating.

If we are having a particularly delicious meal, I'm always tempted to go back for seconds and even thirds.

I've learned a trick that helps me enjoy food to the fullest, while not overeating. Whenever I really want seconds, I first drink a full glass of water. The effects are incredible. Usually in the time it has taken me to drink the glass of water, my brain has had time to register that I am actually full. I almost never go back for seconds.

You can have a glass of water even if you have another beverage. Don't be embarrassed to order water with your soda. You can only gain by having water. There is absolutely nothing to lose.

"But water is boring." If you believe that then spice it up! Have your water with lemon and mint, water with cucumber, water with Texas shaped ice cubes. Have fun with it. Just don't add sugar to it. Treat yourself to a fancy new water bottle. Go ahead: splurge. Install a cold-water tank in your home. Water can only help you and it will make you feel like a million bucks.

Group Discussion Questions:

1. How can you incorporate drinking more water into your life?
2. What unhealthy beverages do you typically drink?
3. What can you do to get excited about drinking water?
4. What other health benefits come from drinking water?
5. When are times you enjoy drinking water?

CHAPTER SIX

GET UNBALANCED

Yoga. Sounds so beautiful rolling off the tongue doesn't it? Words like "zen" and "namus dey" or "haveaniceday" or whatever it is they say. Yoga. That sounds like something I can do! It's just stretching right?!? Wrong. Oh so very, very wrong.

It was a few months after I'd had my fourth child. My core was working over time just to make sure I didn't pee my pants when I laughed. I felt super confident I could take on this "yoga" thing. No problem. Heck, I spend half my life bent over to the ground anyway picking up kids or all the things kids magically put on the floor. I got this.

Ladies and gentlemen, I did not *have* this. Of course I was late to the group exercise class. Like who in the world can be on time with one kid much less four of them. So, lucky me! I got the spot right next to the teacher in the front of the class wickedly close to the giant mirrors. Side note, whoever decided to put mirrors in workout rooms is an evil villain. I jumped right in mid-warm-up. First few moves, no problem. A little downward dog, a little sun salutation. I love this yoga thing! Then come the plank holds. I tell you what, I looked like a baby elephant trying to balance on toothpicks. I would have made Barnum and Bailey's circus proud. About my face; oh Lawd my face! I love how in yoga, everyone is trying to keep this calm and serene face. As if they are not suffering tortuous pain by flexing their muscles in ways they were never meant to go! They are all liars. Liars I tell you. To top it all off? I had rice and beans for lunch just a few short hours before. I'll say no more. I think you get the picture.

We are bombarded by unhealthy eating options and a lightning paced lifestyle. Obesity is now recognized as a public health crisis when historically it was considered a sign of wealth and prosperity. It's a problem that most of America, if not the entire western world is facing. We can't ignore it. We must address it.

Do you feel overwhelmed by all the things you *should do?*

What feels like seconds after your head hits the pillow, you wake up to a blaring alarm clock. Or my personal favorite, a child's voice freakishly close to your face. You rush to get ready for the day, probably skipping flossing because who has time for that? Breakfast is a drive-through down the road where you leave your sunglasses on because it feels like you can hide your shame just a bit more. You barely make it to work on time and are immediately bombarded with a hundred things to do on top of the ones you left from yesterday. You rush out of work, eager to get home to spend time with your spouse, kids or fur babies. You look in your fridge and pantry. They are full, yet somehow there is nothing to eat. You manage to put food on the table, let the dogs out, get some homework done, get the kids to bed, answer an email or three, and crawl into bed to stare at your phone until way later than you intended.

But wait!?! Why didn't you invest in yourself? Workout? Meal prep for the month? Call your mom? Nail that Pinterest project? Invest in friendships? Have a romantic evening with your significant other? Invest in Bitcoin? Take your dogs for a walk? Join the latest network marketing trend that will allow you to have financial freedom and a nice new car?!?

The proverbial "Balance" people speak of is truly an impossibility; quite like my awkward Upward Dogs in yoga. Somehow we have placed our self-worth in our well-balanced achievements. So I say, "To heck with that!"

Get unbalanced.

Just focus on one thing. Invest in your health. Invest in your mental well-being. Stop expecting yourself to be perfect in every area of life. Focus on one thing that is important to you. Try to make one simple change that will change the rest of your life.

You can do everything mediocre, or you can do a few things really well.

Group Discussion Questions:

1. What are your personal priorities? How do you currently invest in these?
2. What things do you need to stop wasting time on?
3. What areas of your life are going well?
4. What areas of your life are hindering your health?
5. What specific things would you like to focus on in your health journey?

CHAPTER SEVEN

CONVENIENCE CONVENIENCE CONVENIENCE

Isn't it amazing how inconvenient modern conveniences are? Like when your phone decides to update when you are right in the middle of using Google Maps on your way to an unknown destination? Or when your ringer goes off in a business meeting? Or when the internet decides to throttle when you are in the middle of your Netflix binge? Ain't nobody got time for that.

I used to live right by a Shipley Do-Nuts. If you don't know what that is, just think of crack-cocaine in doughnut form. I had to drive by that glorious temptation every single day. It was torture. The comfort of complex processed filthy carbohydrates was just one shameful drive-though away. Nine out of ten times, I had the courage and logic to just keep on driving. Unfortunately that one out of ten set me back weeks, even months on my health journey.

Take the inconvenient long way home.

Once I realized the damage I was doing to myself, I began to take the long way home. I avoided the temptation altogether by not driving by it. Yes, it would have been convenient if I just magically gained the will power to say no every time. At this point in my life it would have ben easier to sleep on a cactus. Taking the long way home only added three minutes to my drive and another fifty-cent toll. But it saved me pounds of cellulite. Literally pounds of it. Ain't nobody got time for THAT!

Waste Money.

Have you ever used your lack of money as an excuse not to sign up for a workout class? Or start a weight loss program?

I was in a particularly stagnant season of my health journey. I needed help. I had a good friend who was a professional health expert. I really wanted to ask her to help me make a meal plan, but I was low on cash. You see, I really believe in paying people what they are worth and honoring the hard work they put into getting their degrees. So I didn't want to ask her to help me for free just because we were friends.

I couldn't believe how difficult it was for me to part with a few measly dollars or ask for help! Especially considering this kind of investment would last a lifetime. Not to mention, getting healthier would save me thousands of dollars in health costs down the road if I started taking better care of my body.

So go ahead and waste money. Waste money on health plans, waste money on exercise equipment, waste money on anything that might give you one more minute of health and success rather than fat failure.

You think you can't afford to do it. The reality is: you can't afford NOT to do it. No one dying of heart disease or diabetes in a hospital looks back on their life and goes, "Man, I sure am glad I didn't spend money on that gym membership!"

1. What conveniences are destroying your health?
2. How can you address those issues?
3. What investments in your health have you been hesitant to make because of time or money?
4. What investments have you made in your health journey that have been successful?
5. How will you get your friends and family to honor your inconvenient lifestyle?

CHAPTER EIGHT

HOW DO YOU WANT IT?

I perfectly take care of my health: when I am alone. Which is never. So how do we navigate the world of relationships while so many people bring us down?

I was in my early thirties when I went out to eat with my parents. We went to Olive Garden, the home of the 3000-calorie pasta. Luckily, a friend had introduced me to the unlimited soup and salad combo on the menu on a previous occasion. So I found a hearty vegetable soup that I loved and a salad that is to die for. So I ordered the never-ending soup and salad again while dining with my parents.

My dad immediately chimes in, "That's not all your gonna eat? Is it?" Um, yes dad, it is. It's NEVERENDING food?!? I literally could not have ordered a larger portion option. So then my mom orders a meal that comes with asparagus. She won't touch asparagus with a ten-foot pole. I mean, its green AND it's a vegetable, so no way Jose. Well, I offer to eat some of it so she allows the asparagus to come to the table. We have a delightful meal. I treat myself to some of the asparagus then I push it away. My father instantly chimes in: "You need to eat all of the asparagus."

I thought to myself, "Dad, I'm thirty years old!! If I don't want to finish my asparagus with my NEVERENDING salad, I don't have to!" I couldn't believe how invested he was in my eating, even as an adult. On one hand he wanted me to eat vegetables. On the other hand he wanted me to clean my plate at all costs. Isn't he just like all of us? We desperately want to eat healthy things but we are also trapped in unhealthy habits.

It's a miracle I've reached my thirties without diabetes yet.

Listen, I don't blame my parents. We have since had many laughs about that meal. They did the best they could with what they knew. They protected me from as much pain as they possibly could. Now that I'm a mom, I get it. My parenting philosophy is this: I'm going to do the best I can, and then I'm going to pay for my children's counseling!

Take an inventory of your relationships. Some relationships you are stuck with and some relationships you get to choose. Some of these people breath life and encouragement into you. Some people are very destructive. If the relationship is important, but yet destructive, then do the work to change the relationship into something beautiful and encouraging.

Your health journey is birthed from the deepest parts of your nature and your experiences. To entrust this part of you to someone else is a very vulnerable place to be. How can you expect to be encouraged if the people you are bearing your soul to are destroying it?

Ask yourself the following questions about the people in your life:

- Does this person encourage me or discourage me? Why?

- Do I have open and respectful communication with them?
- Can I share my needs openly?
- Am I encouraging to this person? Can I do this better?
- Can I improve my relationship with this person?

The last question might be the most important. We cannot change people who do not want to change. However, we can improve relationships that have a foundation of mutual love and respect. Some difficulties in relationships can be fixed. Some cannot.

Create healthy boundaries with people AND with food. Honestly, this is one of the solutions to most interpersonal issues. We have a finite amount of energy and time to invest in our health journey. Choose wisely who you seek for encouragement. For the people in your life whom you are stuck with, teach them how to encourage you. If they cannot, then create physical or emotional boundaries that protect you from their poison.

"Boundaries" is a beautiful life-giving word. For example, you don't have to give up brownies completely; you just have to have boundaries with brownies. For some of you, giving up brownies forever is not a very big deal. For others, it would be easier to cut off your pinky toe. Would you believe me if I said there was a way you could eat brownies, stay thin, and not feel any guilt? It is absolutely possible, with *boundaries*.

Having one brownie a month won't make you feel rotten. Eating half the pan, or the whole pan, will destroy you physically and emotionally. It will spike our blood sugar and mess with our hormones. That kind of eating is detrimental to our psychological health.

Extreme food habits lead to extreme health issues.

I was starving one beautiful Saturday evening. It had been a really busy day. I managed to get in a twenty-minute workout so naturally I needed 24,395 extra calories to make up for my expended energy. By the time we finally got home for supper it was a leftovers buffet. After having four babies in six years, I have learned to eat my supper faster than you can say Constantinople. Any of you parents out there totally get it. This particular mealtime went something like this: get the food on the table, get the milk, and then, oh no, not milk, my three year old can't stand milk all of a sudden, so I get the water, and the napkin, and the dropped spoon, and the "mommy sit by me" "no sit by me mommy" so I move my chair to the middle of the room so I am exactly the same amount of centimeters away from each child... I finally get to sit down and eat. I have exactly 1.67 minutes before the baby starts screaming and my mealtime is over. I finished my meal in record time.

The problem with eating this fast is that my body has ZERO time to register food and even less time to decide if I've had enough food. Holy cow did I want my kid's leftover hotdog. So I ate it. I really wanted her uneaten mango also. That's when a miracle happened! I set a boundary with food and I stopped eating. This is the moment where the tide turns.

Boundaries.

In these moments, it literally feels painful to say no to what you want. It reminds me of my last-born child. My precious one-year-old daughter goes into a full-blown temper tantrum if I set her down for even a hot second. Not getting what you want is H A R D. But it is an essential part of life. Ultimately, when you set this kind of boundary on yourself, it leads to freedom.

You see, if I had kept eating, I would have spent the rest of the evening feeling gross and uncomfortably full. All I would've seen in the mirror was the weight I needed to lose. Instead, I endured a few seconds of self-control, and felt confident, successful, and healthy the rest of the evening. You know the best part? I had mango for breakfast the next day totally guilt-free.

Group Discussion Questions:

1. Who is the most encouraging person in your life when it comes to your health?
2. Does social media help you or hurt you?
3. When do you find it difficult to exercise boundaries with food?
4. Who do you need to teach how to encourage you in your health journey?
5. What are some boundaries you need with people? With food?

CHAPTER NINE

HOW DOES IT FEEL?

I've been thinking about my answer to "How did you do it?" I've lost fifty pounds... four times. Most importantly, I've learned how to live so that I can experience the freedom of feeling healthy daily. Sure, I've used a few different programs, 21DayFix by Beachbody, Weight Watchers, keto, etc. But people use those programs all the time and don't actually lose weight. Or even worse, they lose the weight and then put it back on once they stop the program. So how did I *really* do it?

The victory all started when I made a commitment to myself to take care of myself. It had been awfully difficult for decades. I had a million reasons not to invest in my health. I told myself I didn't need help. It wasn't a big deal. I didn't want to be selfish by taking time away from my family to exercise. I didn't want to spend money on diet programs...

But I eventually realized I could no longer go down the road of unhealthy habits. It wasn't the life I truly wanted. It was full of fake excuses not to take care of myself. I finally admitted that it was destroying me.

My father spent the last 20 years of his life in and out of hospitals, had numerous surgeries, and eventually died of cancer. It was hell on all of us. It depressed and divided our family. It was rough. I realized a few months after he died that I was headed in the same direction. I didn't want my children or spouse to go through that! I had to make some changes.

By taking care of myself now, I am taking care of my family in the future.

So how do we do this? How do we take care of ourselves now? How do we change our habitually unhealthy lifestyle?

One effective way to change our habitually unhealthy mindset is to replace the lies with the truth. We believe the lie that overeating will satisfy us.

Ask yourself, "What are the results of your choices? How does it feel after you have over-eaten?"

This is probably the #1 way to overcome overeating! Ask yourself how you feel after every time you eat or exercise. For example: you were dying to eat half the pizza. Did it satisfy you? Or do you feel greasy and disappointed in yourself?

You dreaded going for that long walk. Afterwards, weren't you proud of yourself? Wasn't it just a tad bit easier to face yourself in the mirror for the rest of the day?

You chose to order a salad at a restaurant even though you didn't think it would be filling. Did you still feel hungry thirty minutes after the salad? Probably not!

Do you see how post-choice evaluation can help us make better choices in the future? If you realize that a salad is fulfilling, you may be more willing to order it in the future. If you realize that you feel gross after eating fast-food, then you may be more reluctant to order it in the future.

It is so tempting to ignore the negative consequences of our choices. This is one of the ways we avoid shame in our life, although shame is there for a reason. It is your body's own way of helping you survive, helping you thrive! Deny those instincts to be habitually unhealthy. Then you will not only survive, you will thrive.

Group Discussion Questions:

1. Describe a time you felt bad after eating a particular meal.
2. How do you justify overeating?
3. Describe a time you ate healthy and felt satisfied.
4. When have you experienced exercise that made you feel good?
5. How will you remember to do post exercise/eating evaluations?

CHAPTER TEN

DON'T GO TO THE GYM

Grief is a funny bird. In July of 2019, I was going to celebrate my birthday for the first time without my father. For many folks, birthdays without a parent are not a big deal. But for me, I was born on my dad's birthday. It was a huge deal. Every year he would call and tell me I was the best birthday present he ever received. I wasn't going to hear this for the first time in my life. It was a pain that reached the very marrow of my bones.

I had also had my last baby earlier that year. Hormones are a tricky, tricky thing. Some women barely gain any weight when they are pregnant, bless their hearts. They look like someone just put a tiny basketball under their shirt. Then there are women like me: even my dang elbows gained weight. As I was contemplating my upcoming age (an age I had previously considered old until I had reached it myself), my father's death, and the end of my childbearing years that had left so much fat behind, I didn't exactly feel like putting on my boogie shoes to celebrate my birthday.

As I was driving down an old dirt road in Tanzania, I lifted my eyes and saw the towering 5th highest mountain in all of Africa, Mt. Meru. I'd heard of people who had climbed it before. I thought, "Hey, why can't I do that?"

You can do hard things.

I wanted my physical pain to match my emotional pain. I was also longing for the spiritual experience of seeing the world from the top of a 14,967 foot mountain. Everyone said it was "hard but possible." Or at least that's what I heard because that is what I wanted to hear. I called my friend Erica who recently climbed Meru to ask if it was doable. She was out of town. I didn't get a chance to talk to her before I began my ascent.

Day one, two days before my birthday, not so bad. I saw some giraffes, a giant waterfall, and I was good and tired with only one blister. No biggie. Day two, a lot more steep, a few more hours, on the verge of exhaustion, but I made it to base camp and enjoyed some delicious international fried chicken. Day three, peak day, my birthday, my first birthday without my father...

We began our ascent at 11:30 p.m. so we could reach the summit of Mt. Meru in time to watch the sunrise. The sun would rise from behind Mt. Kilimanjaro which you could see in the distance. The beginning of the hike was quite easy as we travelled up a well-marked trail, a wicked deceitfulness of what was to come. Then we began getting closer to the peak. As we hiked along the ridgeline, the path narrowed with a thousand foot drop off on both sides. Then we had to cross sheer rock faces with only a small chain to hold onto. The steepest places had loose tiny rocks that slid every time you took a step. I couldn't believe the treacherousness of this mountain climb!

I've never begged so much for my life in so short a time. By the grace of God, I reached the summit. I got to watch the sunrise over Mt. Kilimanjaro.

I ugly cried. I cried my heart out. I cried for the fear of climbing back down. I cried for the beauty of creation before me. I cried for the loss of my father. I cried for not hearing his voice tell me happy birthday. I sobbed.

I ran into my friend Erica a few days later. I told her how scary it was! She replied, "Yes, it's very dangerous. I definitely would have told you not to do it." Um, thanks. Wish I would have known that a little bit earlier.

Moral of the story: Don't do hard things. Just kidding! Absolutely do hard things.

Exercise feels impossible to many people. But you can do hard things. Celebrate the ways your body likes to move. Maybe you are a Zumba dancing beast. Or maybe you thrive playing golf. If nature walks make you feel alive, do it. Do it often. Maybe you are a champion arm wrestler. Arm-wrestle everyone you know. If you hate getting sweaty, then swim. If you hate running, then ride a bike. If you hate going to the gym, then go on a walk with a good friend or while listening to an audio book.

Don't obsess over what your body looks like. Obsess over what your body can do. Isn't it cool that people can climb higher than some airplanes fly? Isn't it cool that our bodies can float in water? That people can lift more weight than their own bodies weigh?

Celebrate the sounds you hear on a walk. Celebrate the feeling of relaxation after a good hard workout. Celebrate the legacy of physical health you are teaching your family. Don't go to the gym because that's what healthy people do. Do what you love that gets your body moving.

Group Discussion Questions:

1. Is exercising hard for your? Why or why not?
2. What ways can you get your body moving?
3. What hard things have you overcome in your life before?
4. What hard things do you want to do in the future?
5. How can your people encourage you to get moving more often?

CHAPTER ELEVEN

POSITIVE SELF TALK

No catchy tricky title here. This one deserves to be spoken outright.

Positive Self-Talk.

Positive self-talk is using your thoughts to tell yourself that you are worth good choices. Yes, sometimes that means you are worth a celebratory dessert but it also means you are worth a celebratory salad.

This has probably been the darkest part of my health journey. I wonder if it is one of your most depressing areas as well. On the outside, I've always been a confident capable person. But when I looked in the mirror that is not what I saw. I used to see:

- overweight
- unlovable
- big-nosed
- cellulite
- too tall
- big-boned
- incompetent
- setting a poor example for my kids
- fifty pounds too heavy (the fact that my five year old child weighs less than this was not lost on me)
- lazy
- a disappointment to others

Unfortunately, I could go on and on. The first time I learned about positive self-talk, it was so far from my reality that I thought it was a joke. Maybe you feel the same way too? How easy is it to think positively about yourself? Your body?

The basic principle is this:

If you talk to yourself positively, you will make better choices.

If this seems difficult to do, you are not alone. Even people who don't struggle with their weight can find it very difficult to think kindly. Start with something small. Maybe you like the shape of your fingernails? Maybe you can admit you have a wicked fun sense of humor?

Sometimes, before we can think positively about ourselves, we have to undo the damage inflicted on us by someone else. A good place to start is telling yourself that whoever hurt you was wrong. Maybe you need to go to counseling to get to a point where you can say positive things about yourself. Do it.

**You can't heal from it,
if you don't deal with it.**

Another place to start is with the people who love you. Ask your family or friends what they love about you. Ask for personality traits and physical traits. Don't ask people who will use this as an opportunity to cut you down.

I have been working on positive self-talk for over ten years. This is a habit that is worth changing. It will free your heart. It will strengthen your mind. It will build your ability.

Here are some of the things I can joyfully say about myself now. After you read these, write down a few of your own.

- I love helping others.
- I am a relatively positive person.
- I'm never scared to try new things.
- I have hope of what's to come.
- I have dreams for the future.
- I like a lot of things about myself.
- I deserve to take care of myself.
- I am capable of taking care of myself.
- I can set a great example for my kids.
- I can work hard.
- I am capable of changing my unhealthy habits.

Now, when I look in the mirror, I see someone who is working hard. I celebrate.

Group Discussion Questions:

1. What are some of the negative things you say to yourself?
2. What are some of the things you love about yourself?
3. What scenarios do you find it difficult to think positively about yourself?
4. Take a few minutes and have everyone in the group share something positive about each other.

5. Take some personal time to forgive yourself for being so mean to yourself. Then go celebrate with your favorite veggies.

CHAPTER TWELVE

GOOD CHOICES BEGET GOOD CHOICES

I couldn't believe it. I mean, I was the one who said it, yet I couldn't believe the words actually came out of my mouth.

I told my husband, "I'd like to go on a run this morning."

The silence was deafening. He was so quick to hide the shock in his own voice and sweetly said, "Sure babe, I'll watch the kids." Bless his heart. Well, there it was, totally out there hanging in the air.

Now that the words had been said, I had to do it. I justified the torture that was about to occur by saying to myself, "I can just walk. At least I'll have some peace and quiet away from the kiddos." So I went. In the rain. I went running in the rain. It. Was. Awesome.

We live in a rather wooded area in Africa where many men can be found walking along the roads all day. We live in a very misogynistic culture where women should not be heard or even seen. It's not exactly safe to be a woman on this road alone. So running in my tank top and yoga pants was a sight to see, for sure.

Nonetheless, I went running in the rain. A few minutes into my run I was breathing like an elephant dying of pneumonia when I spotted a beautiful young woman. She must have been on her way to work or to church. She was dressed in fancy shoes, and a ktenge (an African patterned skirt that hides a woman's curves). She was trepidatiously staying a safe distance behind a group of young men. As I caught up with her, she looked at me, smiled, and started running with me!

We flew right past those men and as we did I yelled, "Girls rule! Boys Drool!" I have no idea if they understood English. They got the point nonetheless. This wonderful young woman ran almost the entire next mile with me. There was no way I was going to stop and walk. We were both showing our strength and our confidence and we were doing it together. I wonder if she was my guardian angel or if I was hers on that day. I would have missed this sweet moment if I hadn't said those epic fateful words out loud: "I want to go for a run."

It wasn't long after that I decided to sign up for a fun run race. Making the commitment to an upcoming race held me accountable to continue to get some exercise. I also made healthier choices with my food because I didn't want to destroy my good choices with exercise by binge eating sweets. Healthy choices really can have a snowball effect if you let them.

You can't change your entire health history overnight. But you can make one good choice.

Start there.

Group Discussion Questions:

1. When was the last time you felt discouraged in your health journey? What circumstances led to that?

2. Has there ever been a time you made a series of good choices? What circumstances surrounded that?
3. Have you ever achieved a long-term goal? How about regarding your health?
4. Is it easier to make healthier choices with food or with exercise? Why?
5. Are you feeling inspired about any specific healthy choice right now? Please share.

CHAPTER THIRTEEN

RECRUIT HELP

The truth is, we are instinctually pack animals. We do things together. We work together, we live together, we celebrate together. On the reverse side, we also get into trouble together. It's very difficult to get healthy when our pack isn't on the same page of health goals. So what do we do about this? Two things. First:

Find new members of your pack.

My gorgeous and successful sister-in-law invited me to do a Barre exercise class. For those of you who don't know, it's an exercise regime based on the rigorous training of professional ballet dancing. My first thought was, "No way I'm going to sweat in front of a bunch of ballerinas." My second thought was, "Hey! Maybe this will help me look a little more ballerina-ish!" So I went. It was amazing! I mean, I could barely walk for three days afterwards, but it was an incredible workout. My sister-in-law is an official member of my healthy pack. We enjoy eating unique salads together. We enjoy finding exercises we both like and doing those together as well.

Teach your reigning pack members how to help.

I have a dirty rotten confession to make. I realized one day that I hung out with whichever friend would eat a giant greasy cheeseburger with me so I didn't feel ashamed of my caloric intake. Misery loves company. I had one particular girlfriend I would do this with. We will leave her nameless for privacy's sake. I'll just refer to her as my phat phriend. We would devour cheese fries and milkshakes while complaining about our inability to be skinnier. In the moment, it felt great. The after effects were not so great. Truth was, I really didn't want to struggle with my weight. I wanted to be free from that pain! So we had the DTR. Define The Relationship conversation.

I shared with my sweet friend that I really didn't want to destroy my hard work with greasy cheeseburgers. Turn out, neither did she. We made a friendship pack to eat salads together from now on. We still complain together because that's what makes our friendship fun. So we do it over 500 calories instead of 5000.

So make a mental list today of who you want to be on your team. Also make a list of those you need to teach how to help you. Now go for it.

Group Discussion Questions:

1. Who encourages you to achieve your goals?
2. Who inspires you to make good choices?
3. Who praises you when you have made good choices?
4. Who are your phat phriends? Do you have the courage to teach them how to help you?
5. What healthy choice have you been scared to make because of what people will think of you?

CHAPTER FOURTEEN

TELL YOUR PARTNER TO SHUT UP

Let's get one thing straight. I am not a runner. Yes, I do run, or I guess you could call it running. Frequently people walk past me while I run. But I look like I'm running, so I call it running. I am definitely not a naturally inclined athletic runner. I'll tell you why I do it after I tell you why some of my friends don't.

A beautiful young lady that I had the privilege to mentor shared with me that she doesn't like to run or even go on walks because it is too much time to think. About ten minutes into her walk, she is worried about, well, everything. This feeling makes her uncomfortable so she doesn't exercise at all.

Another beautiful friend of mine, one that is so amazing I hope to be just a glimmer of what she is someday, was put off by my encouragement to "recruit help" like I shared in my last chapter. In a short summary, some of the people closest to her had been discouraging, or didn't encourage her in the way she needed to be encouraged. Frankly, we've all been part of a Facebook group that was an epic waste of time. Hahahah, I just laugh to myself when I think about the last Facebook support group I was a part of.

Living in a foreign country, homeschooling was the best option for my kids. I'll tell ya what, I did not spend $150,000 on a law degree to be a stay at home mom. That's a story for another time. I joined a Facebook group called Homeschool Support Group. I thought, "I need support. I homeschool. Cool!" It was so not cool. I posted a question in the group asking about a specific curriculum. I was expecting answers and encouragement. Boy. Was. I. Wrong. I was like a pound of fresh meat thrown to wild dogs. The very first comment I got was "That curriculum is not homeschool. It is school at home." Um, ok. Then, the next comment was, "Yes I agree with the first commenter. That is school at home and you need to read the group description before you post." Well holy cow, I'm so sorry I wasted your time seeking support on your support group.

This isn't a slam on homeschoolers, non-schoolers, un-schoolers and the likes. This is just a perfect example of needing a specific kind of encouragement and literally getting the opposite. Those women weren't trying to hurt or insult me. They, in fact, needed a very specific kind of support as well. We just weren't a good fit for each other. Just like my beautiful friend, some of the people she hoped would be encouraging to her, couldn't meet her needs.

My husband is one of my biggest supporters. He is also traipsing through my minefield of emotional outbursts, self-deprecating explosions, and sassy retorts.

I had decided to go for a run. I was verbally processing trying to decide how far I wanted to run. My precious husband chimes in and says the death penalty of all motivation to run: "Just go out there and see how you feel." And we are done here folks.

If I based my running goals on how I felt, I would never run at all. Never. So I told him to shut up, in a sweet Southern girl kind of way.

I'm not really advocating using the words "shut up" to your spouse. I am advocating open communication with whoever is in your life. Once my visceral emotional response was finished, I explained to him that for me specifically, I need a goal. Otherwise, I will give up when it feels difficult. He understood. He has never said those daunting words to me again.

Sometimes we don't get to choose an ideal support network. People are just in our lives. So we need to teach them how to support us. Because, let's be honest, we are all a little bit crazy.

Now back to the reason I run. The reason I run, even though I don't always enjoy it, is because I should. We should do hard things. We should press into the thoughts that overwhelm us. We should find peace instead of letting them haunt the recesses of our minds. We should release the endorphins that bring our bodies physical peace while contemplating the "what ifs" that terrify us. We should push through our discomforts.

Think about it: If you could push through your discomforts, would you really have so much to change regarding your health? It is uncomfortable for most of us to make healthy choices. So get uncomfortable. Do the hard thing. Learn that you can. Overcome the feelings that keep you in the bondage of unhealthiness. Press into those dark areas until you find peace. Go running even if you aren't a runner.

1. Do you run? Why or why not?
2. What is a hard healthy choice for you to make?
3. How will you find the courage to make that hard choice?
4. What health goals have you achieved in the past?
5. What hard things have you done before? How did you find the strength? How can you translate that strength to your health?

CHAPTER FIFTEEN

EAT MORE

Did you know there are over 20,000 types of edible vegetables in the world? At least that's what a Google search said so it must be true. I bet you can find a few vegetables you like and a few ways you like to eat them. Do it! Eat more vegetables. Drink more healthy beverages. The more time you spend eating healthy things, the less time you will spend pursuing unhealthy habits.

Replace, don't restrict.

I'll never forget a conversation I had with my gorgeously thin cousin Maggie. She lost weight and has kept it off for years. I asked her how she did it. She starts talking about drinking tea with a drop of coconut oil. At the time, it was the most ridiculous thing I'd ever heard. There is no way drinking tea was going to help me lose weight. I just rolled my eyes and felt angry she was keeping all the juicy secrets to herself.

But over time, I've come to realize she was absolutely correct. She had given me a golden nugget of truth. She replaced unhealthy foods with a healthy beverage that she loved. Instead of shoving chips into her mouth between breakfast and lunch, she would drink a delicious warm cup of tea. She replaced unhealthy food choices with healthy ones: solid gold y'all. Now, I even keep chocolate tea in stock so I drink that instead of eating chocolate from time to time.

Whoever coined the phrase "save room for desert" should be given a thousand wedgies. I hate that guy. I LOVE dessert. There is no need to save room. I will eat dessert no. matter. what. The problem with this saying is that it makes dessert the goal, the prize, the purpose. Don't we agree, the real purpose is to take care of ourselves while enjoying food? How can we enjoy food when we are killing our bodies by eating it? How can we find joy when the second that dessert is gone, we immediately feel disgusted with ourselves?

Our access to dessert has increased one hundred fold. Think about the next month of your life. How many times will you have the opportunity for dessert? Birthdays, holidays, eating out, work meetings, wedding showers, etc. Especially if you are an extrovert, your dessert exposure is unlimited. You have to find a way to keep special things special. Think ahead. If you know you are going to want Talitha's birthday cake on Saturday, then don't get an iced coffee (which is 1% coffee, 97% sugar and 2%milk) on the way home from work. Did you get a slightly sad feeling thinking about having to skip the iced coffee? Me too. So treat yourself instead with something healthier and also delicious. Like frozen grapes. I love eating frozen grapes. Yum yum yum.

If you ate a breakfast that gave you protein to help you concentrate, a lunch that gave you antioxidants, snacks that contained fiber, and a dinner that stimulated your mood long term... you wouldn't have anytime left for detrimental food that destroys your body. You would feel healthier and happier. You would be more satisfied with your body. Every aspect of your life would improve. Don't you want that? Of course you do. So what is one little thing you can start with?

Eat more eggs and bananas.

My body will not let me overeat eggs or bananas. They begin to gross me out after I've had a normal portion. So I "overeat" eggs and bananas because they are healthy foods that I can't actually overeat. What healthy foods are like that for you?

Group Discussion Questions:

1. What foods are healthy that you enjoy?
2. What healthy snack can you joyfully eat instead of your trigger foods?
3. When do you feel most tempted to overeat?
4. When do you feel most confident to make a healthy choice?
5. What is one little change you will make this week to achieve your health goals?

CHAPTER SIXTEEN

DO WHAT YOU LOVE

Of course the universe had to give me a professional dietician as a best friend.

[Cue giant eye roll]

Back in the day when I was in shape, I would always ask her to go running with me and she would always ask to go on a walk. At this point in my life I saw no point in walking. I mean, if the weather was cool enough you wouldn't even break a sweat! What's the point in that?

The point was, instead of drinking beer and sitting on a couch chatting with my bestie, I was moving while talking, and loving every second. Just after my fourth pregnancy and seventy pounds to lose, I fell in love with walking. Running hurt. And walking? Walking is wonderful. You can really think about life instead of just focusing on keeping pace. You can have a wonderful conversation with a friend. You can really listen to the lyrics of your new favorite song. You can be seen in public afterwards without needing a serious shower first. I have learned to love walking. So I do it. Often.

So many times we are defeated before we even begin. Yes, I would love to be an ironman athlete, or a beach body goddess. However, what it takes to get there is impossible for me in this season of life. Going for walks isn't. Doing a thirty-minute workout video isn't impossible either. I can still get results that way. Stop overeaching and defeating yourself before you even start.

Maybe you love to turn the lights down low and throw on some Beyoncé to shake your booty? Then do it! Totally counts.

Focus on what your body can do, not what it looks like.

Here are some ideas of ways to move that you might enjoy:

- walking
- running
- dancing
- bicycle riding
- mountain hiking
- swimming
- water aerobics
- barre method
- workout videos
- yoga
- pilates
- martial arts
- horseback riding
- sit down aerobics
- rock climbing
- cardio gym machines
- group fitness classes
- weight lifting
- pushups before bed
- nature hikes

- basketball
- netball
- baseball
- kickball
- soccer
- rugby
- ultimate Frisbee
- any other group sport
- roller skating
- roller blading
- roller derby
- mall walking
- parkour
- mowing the lawn with a push mower
- gardening

Some of these suggestions probably sent your body into a fight or flight response. Rock climbing does that for me. It's not just a "no," it's a "heeeeeeck no." But others, many others were actually kind of exciting to think about. I'm looking forward to trying a few.

Group Discussion Questions:

1. What are the ways you love to move?
2. What are the fruits, vegetables and proteins that you love to eat?
3. What new ways of exercising will you try?
4. How will you add these activities to your life?
5. Who would do it with you?

CHAPTER SEVENTEEN

REALISTIC EXPECTATIONS
GOALS AND GRACE

When people finally started noticing I was losing weight, I was excited to hop on the scale! I had been working so hard. I started walking again. I was trying a keto diet as best as I could. I would occasionally do twenty minute workout videos with my neighbor. I had been at it hard core for weeks! So I stepped on the scale to see my glorious reward. I had only lost 1.5 pounds. I was devastated. My friend gave me that "muscle weighs more than fat" garbage and it just left me even more discouraged. I didn't workout for a week after that. I had an unrealistic expectation of how quickly I would be able to lose weight. I mean heck, I could put on five pounds in one week if I lived near my favorite fast food restaurant. Why did it take so much effort for such little results? Sigh.

Since when did a number on the scale become the single factor in determining my success? It does not. In fact, it almost always leads me back down the road of self-loathing and the lack of courage to take care of myself.

Celebrate your hard work. Eventually, over time, the results will follow.

When I think about how much my body improved over those few weeks of working out (being able to do pushups, picking up my children without feeling like I was pulling a muscle), I felt a thrill inside! That feeling made me want to work even harder. Maybe your realistic expectation is to make one healthy decision this week. That's a beautiful start. When you achieve that, celebrate in a healthy way. Then, make another achievable goal, a realistic goal.

We all want to be the person that eats exactly the right amount of calories and works out every day. That's totally possible, I mean, unless you have a life. Don't let that get you down!

So often when we don't achieve our perfect scenario, we give up. Which is counter-intuitive. Giving up will definitely not get the results you want for your health! So don't give up!

Goals and grace have a symbiotic relationship. You will get nowhere without goals and you will give up without grace for yourself.

Group Discussion Questions:

1. What makes you angry about your health?
2. What excuses do you make not to exercise?
3. What are three expectations/goals you can give yourself that you are confident you will achieve?
4. How will you bounce back and find motivation after your next health failure?
5. What do you need to forgive yourself for?

CHAPTER EIGHTEEN

MAKE EXCUSES

The person who first said, "there is no crying over spilled milk" has obviously never had a milkshake. I can neither confirm nor deny that I have cried over a spilled milkshake. Lord knows my kids have!

Your body will fight to maintain its comfort level. It is one of our instinctual survival skills. If we create habits that we don't have to think about, then our brains have space for new information. Have you ever driven from home to work and not remembered the drive? If you have driven long enough, then much of driving is achieved in the subconscious. The same is true for our eating habits.

So much of our existence is lived in the subconscious. It is necessary to function in life. We can't be alert and intensely thinking about every single decision. It would be impossible at some point to take in new information. So our incredible brains throw it back to the subconscious: where habits live.

Your instincts repeat behaviors that commonly occur to you. For example, what you order at a restaurant, who you call when you are upset, your normal eating times, what foods you think you like... Here's the good news: you can continue to live in your subconscious habits. That is, if you want nothing to change.

You wouldn't be reading this book if you didn't want something to change. So how do you do it?

It's as simple as 123. Notice I didn't say it's as "easy" as 123? Nothing about this is easy. In fact, going from a habitually unhealthy lifestyle to a healthy one is like a professional boxer learning to go back for more fight when they are on the verge of passing out. For some of you it would be easier to run into a burning building than to change your health habits. You have to find that courage every day, multiple times a day, for the rest of your life. That's hard. But it is not impossible.

First, take an inventory of your unhealthy habits. Is it sodas? Is it eating when you are sad/tired/bored? Is it indulging when there is something to celebrate? You cannot change what you are unwilling to recognize.

Second, apply an outside force. A basic principle of physics: A body at rest will remain at rest unless an outside force is applied. You will continue to be unhealthy if you don't apply an outside force. So what outside force are you going to choose? Are you going to work on your mental health? Find an exercise group? Learn more about your diet through a healthy food program?

Third, try. You cannot be healthier if you do not try. You can be healthier if you try. The only guarantee of failure is when you fail to try. So just do something. Anything. Something is better than nothing. Cliché I know, but true nonetheless.

Go ahead and list every excuse you use for making unhealthy choices. Here are some of my favorites:

I'll deal with it later.

It could be worse.

I missed breakfast so now I can have a 5,000 calorie lunch.

Oreos are cheaper than salad.

I'm not even going to think about how many calories are in this food.

I'm not as fat as some people.

I don't eat fast food that much.

I haven't had doughnuts in a long time.

It's a holiday!

If our economy drops out I can live off my body fat for at least a few months.

I don't like the way healthy food tastes.

I'm too tired to exercise.

The box has "fruit" in the name so it must be healthy.

I'll be hungry again if I eat a salad.

I can't afford these weight loss/fitness programs.

I don't want to.

I don't feel like it.

It's too much effort.

I can't.

It won't make a difference in my life.

I've tried before yet here I am unhappily overweight.

We will all probably die in a nuclear war soon anyway, I may as well enjoy my food now.

Now that we got that out of our systems, let's take another look at those excuses and think them through. Let's find reasons to turn excuses into examples of healthy living. I'll do a few for you.

"I'll deal with it later." You should start now! It will only be harder later. It will actually be easier if you start now.

"It could be worse." You are right. It will be worse if you don't start taking charge of your health.

"I missed breakfast so now I can have a 5,000 calorie lunch." You actually jacked up your metabolism by skipping breakfast and your body probably wants to store all your calories as fat so you better make a healthy choice.

"Oreos are cheaper than salad." I got nothing on this one. #truth

"I'm not even going to think about how many calories are in this food." You already know. Furthermore, you will feel ashamed when you are done. So think about them. Make a healthier choice instead. Drink some water and then get right back to kicking your butt into a healthy place.

Group Discussion Questions:

1. What are some of your unhealthy habits?
2. What excuses do you make for overeating?
3. What "outside force" will you apply to your life?
4. How will you try to do better?
5. Who can help hold you accountable to your efforts?

CHAPTER NINETEEN

MY CHEESEBURGER SALAD

One of the oldest texts in the world, so old it was passed down orally before it was ever written, puts our struggles on blast. This guy in the story named Job said, "Don't people complain about unsalted food? Does anyone want the tasteless white of an egg? My appetite disappears when I look at it; I gag at the thought of eating it!" Me and Job would have been homies back in the day.

I hated salads with a passion: unripe tomatoes and soggy lettuce. Yuck. I swore I would never eat salads. So my dietician best friend responded with, "Challenge accepted." As I was on a walk with her one day I was complaining about salads. She asked why I hated salads so much. Let's be real: because cheeseburgers just taste better.

Fast forward to the freakin weekend. She asked me to hang out and have a girls night out on the town. We began the evening at a well known restaurant in the Houston area. Did you know Houston is one of the "fattest" cities in the world? H-town represent! That's because Houston has AMAZING food. Talk about taste-bud titillations! We sat down at a super fun booth with pure white napkins and a flower centerpiece. I'm drooling, literally, over the five course meal I'm about to throw down, when she drops the fatal news on me.

"I brought you here so you can try one of their salads. They are divine." Well adios bestie, I'll see ya next lifetime. Ha, not really.

I tried the salad; and I loved it.

She then took me to a few different restaurants where the salads were really delicious. I realized I liked them ok. The next obstacle for me was to desire them over a cheeseburger. Inconceivable!

She slapped me with this cold hard truth:

Stop expecting a salad to taste like a cheeseburger.

You see, I could never appreciate a salad as long as I was comparing it to my favorite greasy meal. Nevertheless once I looked at the health benefits of a salad, once I appreciated it for what it was, I began to desire them *instead* of cheeseburgers. Because, at times, I desired my health more than I desired a taste-bud explosion.

Have you ever heard of a litmus test? It's this little piece of paper that you place into a liquid. The piece of paper changes color to determine the acidity of the liquid. One definition of a litmus test is: a decisively indicative test. So what does this have to do with your health?

Think about a food that you have never craved but don't hate. For me it would be something like cucumber, papaya, plain rice...Whatever you come up with will be your litmus food. Now, the next time you really want to eat something, ask yourself, if this *something* was my litmus food, would I still want to eat?

This is one way you can determine if you are really hungry or not. If my litmus food was Oreos, I'd never stop eating. Sometimes we cannot tell the difference between hunger and desire. Hunger doesn't get us into trouble. Desire does. So find a food that you don't feel tempted to overeat. That can be your litmus food. If that food sounds good to you, then you are probably hungry. If your litmus food doesn't sound appetizing to you, then you might be emotionally eating. You should strongly reconsider whether to eat or not.

So what do you do now that you have determined that you really are hungry? Rate your hunger on a scale from 1 to 10. One means, "If I eat another bite I won't be able to swallow" and ten means "I could eat my pinky finger if I added ketchup."

Always start with protein.

Dish yourself a fist size of food of everything except vegetables. You can eat as many vegetables as you want. I know what you're thinking and the answer is no. Spinach inside a vat of oily melted cheese does not count as a vegetable. I'm talking about real non-processed veggies. Once you finish this serving, wait thirty minutes. If you are having difficulty waiting, then drink an entire glass of water. Now, after thirty minutes, re-evaluate your hunger scale. If you need to eat more, then eat something without processed sugars. Try to find something with protein, fiber or nutrients.

Group Discussion Questions:

1. Do you enjoy salads? Why or why not?
2. What can be your litmus test food?
3. Where are you on the hunger scale right now?
4. How can you add more vegetables to your diet?
5. How can water help you achieve your health goals?

CHAPTER TWENTY

YOU DO YOU

If you are reading this book, and you've read this far, this is probably not the first time you have tried to lose weight or get healthier. Some researchers say that 95% of people who lose weight gain it all back within a year.[1] There is a reason the health and wellness industry is a trillion dollar industry.[2] And since everything we read on the internet is true, wink wink, we are all walking an uphill road, both ways.

I did some intensive therapy in my late twenties. One of the big factors in my emotional healing was identifying my frozen moments. A frozen moment is an experience in your past that shapes the person you are today.

My frozen moments...

I was in the third grade when Jamal Johnson said I looked like Pinocchio. He said my nose was big. To this day I still think I have a big nose and contemplate a nose job.

I was twelve the first time I realized I had cellulite on my thighs. I was probably 5'8" by this point. My very best friend was a voluptuous 5' flat without an ounce of cellulite on her body. Unfortunately at twelve, the girls are growing faster than the boys. So naturally all the

---

[1] http://www.nytimes.com/1999/05/25/health/95-regain-lost-weight-or-do-they.html
[2] https://www.globalwellnessinstitute.org/press-room/statistics-and-facts/

boys wanted to date my tiny friend instead of the amazon I was becoming.

I was sixteen the first time I was officially categorized as overweight.

I was eighteen the first time my dad went to the hospital for chest pains and heart disease.

I was nineteen the first time I lost fifty pounds.

I was twenty-one the first time I ordered a salad as a meal.

I was twenty-nine when my doctor told me I was gaining too much weight with my first pregnancy.

I was thirty when I began begging God to help me be free from the weight: the weight on my body, the weight on my emotions, the weight on my confidence, the utterly devastating weight of self -loathing.

I was thirty-one when I lost 60 pounds... the second time.

I was thirty-two when I gained 70 pounds with my second pregnancy.

I was thirty-six when my father died after 20 years of heart disease, diabetes and cancer.

These moments are just the tip of the iceberg that created an unmotivated overweight version of myself. Some others are just too intimate to share.

Since therapy, I've recognized my frozen moments that have held me back from achieving my health goals. I have been intentional to deal with them and heal from them. I am thirty-seven-and-a-half and finally feeling the freedom of the healthy life style I've been longing for my entire life. I have lost the weight I wanted to and I am maintaining a healthy life.

What are your frozen moments? Challenge yourself to talk about these. Go through them deeply with a counselor or an encouraging friend. Find the truth in them. You did not deserve the abuse. You are not a victim of your upbringing. You can choose to live differently. You are capable of working hard. You can be free from the despair.

How do people break free from the pain of the past? They make a commitment to themselves to do whatever it takes to break free. I made a commitment to myself.

There were many failures. There were many ugly cries. I committed to never giving up. I committed to picking myself up off the floor after each failure. I committed to trying things I'd never tried before. I committed to learn new things.

So make a commitment to yourself. Commit to taking care of yourself.

That's it. Raise your right hand, and repeat after me:

I, state your name, do hereby solemnly swear, I will love myself, even if I feel like no one else loves me. I will celebrate my body by giving it effective fuel. I will move around in ways that bring a smile to my face, eventually. I will forgive myself on the days I don't. I will encourage others to care for themselves as well. I will find "my people" who will encourage me toward health. I will not obsess over unattainable results. I will celebrate every ounce of hard work toward my goals. I will not punish myself for my failures. I will learn from them. I can do hard things. I will do hard things.

Group Discussion Questions:

1. If you are able to, please share some of your frozen moments.
2. What food habits did you have as a child?
3. How can you heal from your frozen moments?
4. How can you use your frozen moments to find motivation to be healthier?
5. Say the commitment statement together as a group. What do you think about it?

CHAPTER TWENTY ONE

GET SICK

So, I started keto last week. I'm already down two pounds! It may be because of a nice African virus that caused an "everything must go sale" but I'll take it either way. So get sick! Not the African virus kind of sick, but the "I'm a badass and I'm going to kick ass" kind of sick. (If you are offended by my use of the word "ass," please forgive me for my asinine rhetoric. You may change the sentence to "I'm amazing and I'm going to do amazing things.")

I'm not advocating for keto specifically. I chose keto because of in depth research, friendly inspiration, and the all you can eat avocado buffet. There are literally thousands of ways to get healthy. Try some of them (doctor approved of course).

Become a Lifetime Learner.

The easiest way to learn something is to love what you are learning. For reasons I'll never understand, my husband LOVES documentaries. Because of it, he continues to amaze me with his knowledge and wisdom on the most obscure topics. I, on the other hand, am extremely extroverted. The most progress I have ever made in my health journey was finding people I wanted to learn from, and befriending them. Find what works for you, and never stop learning. Here are a few suggestions of ways to continue learning about your health:

1. Documentaries
    a. Fast Food Nation
    b. Super Size Me
    c. Fat Sick and Nearly Dead
    d. Food, Inc.
    e. Forks over knives
    f. etc.
2. Books
3. Weight Watchers
4. Food tracking apps like LoseIt
5. Beach Body
6. Overeaters Anonymous
7. Magazines
8. Gym Memberships
9. Social Media
    a. Join a group or follow someone who is posting health and wellness tips
    b. Don't do this one if you already struggle with setting limits on your screen time. There are plenty of other ways to learn about your health that won't lead to destructive patterns in your life.
10. Personal Trainers
11. Cooking classes
12. Freezer Meal Parties
13. Nutritionists

If there was anything in that list that sounded interesting to you, go for it. Start looking for the next opportunity. You do you.

Group Discussion Questions:

1. What ways have you learned about your health in the past?
2. What is something you enjoy that also teaches you more about health?
3. What new ways can you look for healthy education?
4. How will you find the time to add a new learning avenue to your life? What can you let go of to make that happen?
5. How can you put your knowledge into action? What obstacles must you overcome?

CHAPTER TWENTY TWO

BEWARE OF THE MARKETING MONSTER

"RAISES METABOLISM"
"ORGANIC"
"POST MENOPAUSAL SUCCESS"
"NO GMOS"
"NATURAL"
"FAT BURNING"
"50% LESS FAT"
"ELIMINATION DIETS"
"GUARANTEE"
"LOSE 30 POUNDS"

Just because someone somewhere lost weight on a certain meal plan doesn't mean you need to go all in. Most quick weight loss plans end disastrously. If you lose the weight, the probability of putting it all back on is likely. Why is that? Because nothing in your habitual lifestyle changed. I heard some crazy statistic that 90% of all people who lose more than 10 pounds gain it all back within a few months. So you basically end up where you started with a little more weight and a whole lot of defeat.

Remember those advertisements in the 1900's that said cigarettes gave relief to people with asthma, cough, bronchitis, influenza and shortness of breath? Looks can be deceiving my friends.

But wait right there, Charlie Goodnight! Didn't you just tell us to try all of those programs?

Yes I did. Yes I did. I still stand by that. Because each time you try something new, you learn. You learn what new foods you enjoy. You learn that adding a side of fries adds 700 calories. You learn what changes are difficult for you. You learn what improvements you can keep. You are making progress. Progress should be celebrated.

One of the biggest advertising lies is "healthy food." Did you know the word "natural" can legally be used to describe anything? Literally everything comes from our natural surroundings. Toilet cleaner? Natural. Granola bars? Natural. Roach spray? Natural.

One particularly damaging claim is "50% less fat." Which probably means they made up for the difference with artificial sweeteners. Healthy fats are not bad for you. Sugar turns into fat in your body when you eat more than your body needs day to day, which is shockingly little. You can even get too much sugar from eating too much fruit! If you have more questions about this, please ask a professional to explain the glycemic index.

So how do you know what foods to buy? A good rule of thumb is to choose the perishables. Stay on the outside aisles of the supermarket: vegetables, fruits, dairy, meats... The more vegetables and protein you get in your diet, the easier this whole "healthy living" thing becomes. If it has a long shelf life, it will probably make your butt so big you could use it as a shelf. Just sayin.

Knowledge is power.

Group Discussion Questions:

1. What advertising claim have you seen lately that was absurd? Doesn't have to be health related.
2. What perishable foods do you enjoy eating?
3. What processed foods will be hard to let go of?
4. What are some ways to prepare vegetables that you enjoy?
5. Have you ever read ingredient labels? What has surprised you?

CHAPTER TWENTY THREE

USE TOOLS, DON'T BE ONE

If you are in the profession of helping people make healthier choices, this chapter is for you. One purpose of this book is that it would be encouraging to those who are struggling day to day to live a healthy confident lifestyle. Another goal is to give health professionals, dieticians, personal trainers and the likes some insight into how to help their clients and patients think differently.

During my second pregnancy I gained 70 pounds. It was a combination of a lifetime of unhealthy habits, the stress of starting a law firm, being pregnant while having a one year old, and living near a legion of fast food restaurants. I worked so unbelievable hard and lost fifty pounds after that pregnancy. I was still twenty pounds overweight.

So as I entered my third pregnancy, I wanted help. I did NOT want to gain 70 pounds again! I got a referral from my doctor to speak with a dietician about maintaining a healthy weight gain during pregnancy. I met with a hospital dietician. I was so excited! First, she took my height and age. Next we sat down to have a discussion. I'm about three months pregnant at this point. I'll never forget the next thing that came out of her mouth. She told me my goal weight should be 140 pounds. Perhaps you remember from a previous chapter that my body type is more of an amazon than a ballerina?

Sure, I can weigh 140 pounds... If I cut off my left leg. I haven't weighed that little since I was 10 years old. Let me tell you what, I did NOT leave that meeting feeling motivated about my health. I left feeling super depressed and feeling like I was doomed to obesity for the rest of my life. You see, she was a tiny little young thing who had clearly never had to lose more than ten pounds in her life. She has this cute little dietician formula that spit out caloric meal plans and goal weights. So that's what she did—and it destroyed me. She meant well, but she literally achieved the opposite of what her goal was.

"Diet and Exercise" say the experts. It is not just diet and exercise. We have all heard that a million times. So for the love of God stop saying it. It is not working. It is so much more than that. It is stress, it is childhood trauma, it is psychological pain, it is addiction, it is confidence, it is a lack of knowledge. It is so much more than "diet and exercise" and a stupid little scale that doesn't take into account genetics and hip size.

Many people refuse to participate in programs like Overeaters Anonymous or Weight Watchers because of the identity that comes with it. I urge you, don't deny yourself excellent help because of some social stigma. For years I shunned Weight Watchers because I never wanted to admit to myself that I was overweight. "It's just baby-weight, I'm just getting older, guys like big butts and they cannot lie..." But by the grace of God, some family and friends that I love dearly, who weren't nearly as vain as I, joined the program and had great success! I swallowed my pride and joined also.

I learned valuable tools that I will carry with me the rest of my life. I felt free. I felt progress. I felt encouraged. My pride only made me embarrassed to look in the mirror. My surrender brought me one step closer to freedom.

A tool is someone who refuses to try something that could help them because of their image. A tool is a health professional who thinks its just as simple as "diet and exercise." Don't be a tool, you fool. To think you don't need help is like a person trying to cut their grass with only their hands. There are so many tools out there to help you on your health journey.

Group Discussion Questions:

1. What tools have you used to help you on your health journey?
2. Is there a time when you sought help from a professional and you left discouraged?
3. Have you ever had an experience with a health tool and felt encouraged?
4. What prevents you from moving forward with a new avenue of health?
5. How can you overcome these excuses?

CHAPTER TWENTY FOUR

STRESS MANAGEMENT

It was one of those days. The day started out nicely actually. I had brunch with a good friend; the weather was crisp, cool, and sunny. The kids did beautifully with homeschooling. In fact, I was so on top of the world I even encouraged my husband to leave me alone with the children that evening while he went out with his buds. Then the bewitching hour descended on us like fog on the moors of England. It's that beautiful hour near bedtime where your kids turn into little havoc wreaking gremlins with the sole mission of destroying you.

I was going about my business video recording all of my children's impromptu dining room dance shows and violin practices. I casually took the baby for a bath because it was her bedtime. My oldest daughter walks in and angrily throws a picture at me that she drew. It said "mom" with a drawing of me crying that she crossed out about a hundred times.

Apparently, she was not finished performing her violin solo and I was the most "terrible person in the world." Honestly, it broke my heart. The next thing I know, my seven year old is picking up my five-year-old by the neck because she thinks she is the Greatest Showman's trapeze artist. I'm yelling, they're all crying. Glory be. So naturally I ate chocolate for dinner. Stress overload. It didn't help. It just made me feel bad about myself.

A few years ago I met a wonderful woman who had a rockin body. She shared with me that she didn't really have the energy to get into shape until her last child was three years old. Hear me on this folks, I'm not saying put off your health until your life is less stressful because, let's be honest, that day may never come. I *am* saying:

Use healthy choices to help manage your stress.

Maybe your stress level is so intense that the most you can muster is adding a side of veggies to your pizza. Or driving to the gym to eat a cheeseburger in the parking lot and driving home. I can neither confirm nor deny that I actually did this. Hey, at least I went to the gym! It's all about building healthy habits people. Don't judge.

Using exercise to manage your stress is extremely helpful to your mood stability. It will help you sleep better at night. It will help regulate your moods. It will help your mind work more sharply and effectively. Cut yourself some slack in difficult seasons. Love yourself with healthy choices and positive self-talk. Also, give yourself a break from unachievable goals. Make small bite sized goals. They say you can eat an entire whale—if you take it one bite at a time. I wonder what whale tastes like? I digress. The point is: make small achievable goals. Annihilate them, and then make more.

Group Discussion Questions:

1. What will be your next small achievable goal?

2. What stress are you fighting in your life right now?
3. What healthy stress management techniques do you use?
4. What unhealthy stress management techniques do you suffer from?
5. What will be your next small achievable goal after you master the goal in question number one?

CHAPTER TWENTY FIVE

DRINK POISON: BE RUDE

I swear to you, the first time you try apple cider vinegar, it will absolutely taste like you are poisoning yourself. It's much like the first time you taste beer. You think, why in the world would anybody choose to drink this garbage? But they do. Furthermore, unlike beer, apple cider vinegar has some great health benefits.

It was a long day of social engagements. A friend was having a tea and clothing sale. Our neighbors invited us over for a "brie." That's South African for Bar-B-Que. Both parties were serving alcohol. Somehow they both chose rosé as their beverage of choice. Both of these relationships were relatively new and I didn't want to offend. I didn't want to disappoint. I didn't want to spoil anyone's fun. So I drank it. Gross.

Who in the world likes rosé?!? It tastes like a sippie cup of juice left in a hot car for way too long. So you might ask me, why in the world did you drink the entire glass, not only once, but twice? Because people-pleasing in regards to food had become a way of life: a destructive, disappointing, false life. I wasn't being true to who I was. I was being fake.

Who am I really? I am someone who will offend others if it means I can help someone. I am someone who cares about my body. I am someone who doesn't waste calories on unhealthy food or drinks that I don't like because it is an insult to my taste buds.

Once I realized I had made choices that are counter to what I believe about myself, that's when I rode the lightning and downed the poison: I drank apple cider vinegar. Allegedly, apple cider vinegar has a number of health benefits, including weight loss. I've heard if you drink a teaspoon a day it will regulate your digestive system. So I diluted a teaspoon with as much water as I could get down in one gulp. No way did I want to prolong this crazy form of torture with even two gulps.

It had a two-fold effect on me. I began to feel free again. I had taken my health back into my own hands. I no longer made decisions based on the whims of others. I cared about my body and I was going to make healthy choices for it.

It also felt a bit like punishment (*see above description of apple cider vinegar). Now people, if we find out in a few years that apple cider vinegar causes some sort of cancer, then by all means do not try this at home. Don't do it just because I told you to do it. That is exactly the kind of psychological pressure that led me to drink crapé, I mean rosé. Get into the habit of only eating and drinking what you want to eat and drink for your health goals. Who cares what other people think? Will they be there to hold your hand when you are dying of cancer? Will they be there to help you up the curb because your diabetes-ridden feet can't quite budge that heavy load? Their emotional manipulation isn't a reason to destroy your life. You do you.

Make an inventory of the people, places, and scenarios where you struggle to make healthy decisions. Here are a few of mine:

- Around family. 'Nough said.
- When my hottie husband suggests anything. I'm so distracted by his handsomeness I'm just putty in his delicious hands.
- When I want to "go with the flow."
- Every time pizza is around.
- Houston Livestock Show and Rodeo. Can we say fried oreos and funnel cake people!?!
- Potlucks
- A 150 mile radius of Shipley's doughnuts

It wouldn't be uncommon for all or most of those things to happen in the same month. If I didn't deny my instincts to enjoy food or go with the flow, I'd have eaten seven-unwanted-pounds worth of calories in a simple month. Do you know what seven pounds of fat looks like? Google it. I'm sorry and you're welcome.

Group Discussion Questions:

1. What scenarios do you find it difficult to make healthy choices?
2. When do you find it easy to be successful with healthy choices?
3. Who influences you in a negative way? A positive way?
4. Brainstorm ideas with each other to combat those difficult scenarios. Remember, what works for you doesn't necessarily work for someone else. So don't give advice. Just share experiences.

5. Choose a re-set button for your health. For me, it was apple cider vinegar. It can also be eating a salad or fasting for one meal. What will your re-set be?

CHAPTER TWENTY SIX

GIVE UP

Give up punishing yourself because you are not

___________________ (fill in the blank).

No, you aren't a high school athlete who can put down an entire Papa Johns pizza as an appetizer and still have zero body fat. No, you aren't running a ten-minute mile or lifting fifty-pound dumbbells. No, you aren't fitting into your pre-baby clothes (moms AND dads, can I get an amen?!?). No, you aren't at your goal weight and haven't been for a very long time, if ever. No, you don't want to see yourself in pictures. This is the cold hard truth. However, this is not the end. It is the beginning.

Let's be honest with ourselves. Sure, we would love the metabolism and freedom of youth. Or someone else's youth because there are those of us who have never been thin a day in our lives. But it is impossible to go back in time. Wisdom comes from experience. Sure, we can all look back on seasons of our life and rejoice. If you make a commitment to your health, then you can also look toward your future and rejoice.

That's when it finally happened for me.

It was a lazy Sunday. We went out to lunch with some friends. I ordered a salad while everyone else got pizza or authentic Chinese food. Then they wanted ice cream. Every other person, all seven of them got ice cream. I didn't. Let me tell you, it was not exciting. I found myself staring at their ice cream.

My mouth would begin to water. Just one taste, just a small cup; I had a salad shouldn't that mean I earned the ice cream? I worked out a couple of times this week. No one would know. I could workout again later. Everyone else is eating it and they aren't overweight. It's my favorite flavor...

And then I would snap up and look around to make sure no one noticed my adulterous love affair with ice cream. There were many times where I was embarrassed at how I was longingly looking at it. You know what? I don't even like ice cream that much. My food addiction is actually to the adventure of tasting life. I love that exciting feeling of a longing fulfilled: instant gratification at it's finest. Half the time I am looking forward to the experience much more than I am looking forward to the actual food.

Luckily, that particular afternoon, I used positive self-talk to get me through those infinitely tortuous minutes. I told myself, "You are finally starting to lose weight. You are worthy of healthy choices. You have the strength within you to be healthy. Don't throw it out the window. You don't even like ice cream that much. You will absolutely regret it a few minutes later if you eat ice cream." This positive self-talk worked long enough to get me through the temptation. An hour later, when I was reflecting on the day, I felt happy. Normally that was when I would feel ashamed of myself for whatever food choices I had made that day. But not this day! This day, I stood firm. This day, I prioritized myself.

Make short-term sacrifices for long-term goals.

This day, I felt even more motivation to take care of myself. It really is a snowball effect. Good choices beget good choices. I don't think I have ever made that many good choices in a row. It felt amazing. It was like a runner's high, but with food. An eater's high? A fooder's high? A fatter's thigh? Whatever. It was epic.

So give up punishing yourself. Start celebrating every good decision. Did you choose a lower calorie salad dressing? Did you skip the shake? Did you set your alarm to get up a little bit earlier? Did you spend time thinking about how to make better choices? Did you actually make a healthier choice? Amazing. Great work. Keep it up, one bite at a time.

Group Discussion Questions:

1. What do you hate about yourself? How motivated do you feel when you think about it?
2. How can you move on from punishing yourself?
3. What did you love about yourself in the past? What do you love about yourself now?
4. How can you focus more on the things you love about yourself?
5. What victories can you celebrate this week?

CHAPTER TWENTY SEVEN

BE DRAMATIC

There is great power in symbolism. I was asked to speak to a beautiful group of women about insecurity. At first I was offended. Why would they think I had anything to say about insecurity? Do they think I'm insecure? They must think I struggle with confidence. They must think I'm ugly....

Hello insecurity!

As I dove deeply into this topic, I realized that I was still harboring the insults of ten-year-old boys, the cruelty of thirteen-year-old girls, and the disloyalty of boyfriends from long ago. I was a shell of confidence on the outside yet a vapid desolate wasteland of confidence in my mind. Why do we always dwell on the negative? That is a book for another time.

Stop comparing and start celebrating.

Aren't we fascinated by what we can do as humans? Don't we just love to watch grown men sweat and run into each other? Or pretty ladies pretend it doesn't hurt when they dance on their tippy toes? Isn't it cool to learn about incredibly unique thinkers who have created technology that we've never even imagined was possible? We love to enjoy what our bodies can do. So start enjoying what your body and mind can do.

As I explored the topic of insecurity, I realized I still had a lot of healing to do. Instead of acting in response to how much I loathed myself, I wanted to act out of love for myself. I wanted to see the world differently.

So I got my nose pierced.

It was dramatic. I mean, drunk college kids get facial piercings, not a thirty-five year old attorney mom! But it was important for me to do this for myself. It was my Ebenezer: my symbol of a turning point in my life. I about had a heart attack when the piercing artist told me I could not take it out for six months. That will look professional to a federal judge... NOT.

But the most beautiful part: no matter where I'm looking, I can always see the piercing in my peripheral vision. It's like I see the world through a new perspective. It's a constant reminder to me to see the world through my strengths instead of my weaknesses. I took off the burdensome wet fleece blanket of shame and self-loathing and put on an Egyptian cotton gown of freedom and authority over my health.

Group Discussion Questions:

1. What pain from the past is preventing you from a healthier future?
2. Are you willing to make today a turning point in your life?
3. How can you memorialize your new beginning?
4. On a piece of paper make a list of the "old you." As a group, throw away the "old you" lists.
5. On a new piece of paper, make a list of the "new you." This is the person you are, the one you will

strive to be, the healthiest version of yourself. Place the "new you" list somewhere you can see daily. Remember, the old has gone and the new has come.

CHAPTER TWENTY EIGHT

WHAT THE F!

Ahh the F-word. Fat. There, I said it. Gives me all the feels. The "fat" I'm talking about is the fat in our diets: healthy fat. I also love the F-word: fiber. I promise, if you focus on vegetables, fiber, healthy fats, and stay away from sugars, you will feel amazing. Sugar jacks up our hormones. Sugar gives us mood swings. Sugar prevents our bodies from knowing when we are full. Sugar is the real cuss word here.

Its not a coincidence that Fat and Free both begin with the letter F. Actually, that is a coincidence. It's probably the epitome of a coincidence.

One of the biggest problems with fad diets is that we are not replacing unhealthy foods. We are only trying to restrict ourselves. This is not sustainable long term. We need to replace unhealthy foods with healthy ones: foods that help us feel satisfied and full. Have you ever heard the saying, "Don't go to the grocery store hungry." You just end up buying unhealthy food and overeating. Processed carbohydrate-laden foods do nothing to fuel you body.

Food is for Fuel.

I just really love F-words apparently.

For most of my life, food was not fuel. It was a feeling. What did I "feel" like having for dinner? Food helped me escape my emotions. It distracted me from stress. It was a way to have fun. Or so I thought.

The problem is that it was having the opposite effect. I was not feeling great being overweight. I was having detrimental emotions because of irregular sugar spikes. I tell you what: there is no kind of fun like "spilling over your airplane seat into your neighbors seat" kind of fun. I swear they make planes these days for hobbits and not real people. Or when you get in a bathtub and can only put two inches of water because otherwise it spills over the side. Fun times kids. Fun times. Food wasn't freeing me, it was failing me.

I'll be honest, this *"feelings"* relationship with food has not completely gone away. But my conscious mind has conquered those lies that sugary foods will make me feel better. My logical mind desires food that make me feel full; food that fuels my mind and body. Food that makes me feel strong enough to exercise or play with my kids. So remember the F words:

Fuel Fiber Fats Fegetables

It's a word.

Group Discussion Questions:

1. How can you use logic to defeat your feelings that lead to unhealthy habits?
2. If you know a certain food is unhealthy, why do you eat it anyway? What's happening in your mind in that moment?
3. What foods do you enjoy that are good for your body and mind?

4. How can you add more F-word foods to your daily routine?

5. If food is no longer an option to deal with stress or emotions, then what else can you do to deal with stress and emotions?

CHAPTER TWENTY NINE

GET DIVORCED

Get Divorced. Divorce your inner child. Divorce fat mirrors. Divorce your bottom half.

Divorce your inner child. I woke up to a screaming child. She was just mad she was awake. So she screamed. I set her down next to her sister on the couch. So she screamed. We took the ipad away. So she screamed. Holy Moses I feel like I have PTSD from the sheer volume of my kids over the years. Before you go get all judgmental on me, she is only thirteen months old, so no, she can't "use her words" and yes I let her look at pictures on the ipad. Moms are some of the most judgmental people I know. Not elephant mamas though. I love elephants for a few reasons. The entire herd takes care of the mama. Also, they are always fatter than me.

Let's get back to the inner child. Your inner child in this context is that voice that says you need things you don't actually need. Often my inner child feels like I need food that I will regret later. I have a million excuses to eat that food. If you hear your inner child say any of the following, then you need to stop, drop, and roll-out:

- I *feel* like eating __________.
- I exercised today so I can eat __________.
- I've had a hard day so __________ would be ok to eat.
- He's thin and he gets to eat __________.

- I've been eating healthy all week so I deserve ________.
- I'll start eating healthy right after I eat ________.
- I'll only have one small piece of ________.

Stop. Stop that detrimental way of thinking.

Drop. Drop that food into the trash. I don't care if you spent fifty dollars on it. Throw that delicious detrimental food away and then squirt dish soap on it so you don't go back into the trash to get it. Trust me on the dish soap.

Roll. No, don't roll your burrito inside a whipped-cream covered pancake. Dang, that sounds good. Roll your big butt outta there to avoid the temptation! If you're in a restaurant, go positive self talk yourself in the bathroom. Who cares if someone else is in there!

Stop what you are doing immediately, drop the food in the trashcan, and roll away from the temptation. Eating these foods, these trigger foods, will burn you like a wildfire.

I am not saying you can never enjoy savory foods that you enjoy again. I am saying the emotional state under which you have these savory foods is destroying you.

There is a better way.

There is a better way to enjoy the foods you love; a way that feels like freedom; a way that you can enjoy your food without shame and guilt. But it is not this way.

Divorce that emotional relationship with food. **Divorce your inner child.**

I was on a wicked health streak. I mean, the number on the scale was going down, pants were fitting instead of just suffocating my cellulite. I was exercising! So I put on my cutest outfit for a dinner party. I was feeling so confident.

Then, I looked into a full-length mirror at the hostess's house. Not only did this mirror not recognize the few pounds I had lost, but it so graciously added about twenty more. It was a fat mirror. But for the laws against vandalism, I would have given that mirror a piece of my mind. That mirror destroyed me for the rest of the day. You see, my mirror at *home* only shows me from the waist up. That is glorious because I carry aaaaallllll my weight in my lower half. When I look at my mirror at home I feel like me.

Replace your mirrors. I'm not kidding about this. When you see a reflection of yourself, it should make you feel like the confident version of yourself. Maybe that means it's only your rearview mirror for a while. Maybe it's a full length. Maybe it's a mirror on the floor that shows off your amazing legs. I love that radical religious guru who said, "If your right hand causes you to stumble, then cut it off!" Throw away your mirrors. Focus on the visuals of yourself that you love. **Divorce your fat mirrors.**

While you're at it, **divorce your bottom half.** Or maybe, for you, it's your top half. Everyone should have a part of their body that they love. Or maybe, if you are really struggling, a part of your body that you hate a little less than the others. Focus on that part of your body.

Dress in a way that shows off your favorite body parts. Place mirrors strategically so that you feel confident when you look in them. Share with your close friends the parts of yourself that you enjoy and ask them to notice you and be encouraging also. When you workout, punish those other parts of your body. Do the kind of reps that prevent you from sitting on the toilet. When you feel that pain, remind yourself that you are an incredible specimen. You are strong. You overcome.

I am absolutely not advocating for body shame. Saying "focus on the part of your body that you love" does not mean the inverse, "It's ok to hate the other parts of your body." It is not. I confess, this is hard for me to do. So I'm seeking growth in this area of my life as well. So far, I started following some body positivity gurus on social media. I've purchased clothes that are cute even though they do not accent my favorite body parts and I rock them. When I workout, I "punish" these parts so that when I look at them, I see strength instead of failure. We are all works in progress.

I am definitely not talking about divorcing your spouse. In fact, in a previous career, I was a divorce attorney. Side-note, I genuinely believe if people would take the same amount of time and money they spend in a divorce proceeding trying to destroy their spouse, and instead, use it trying to heal their marriage, it would dramatically decrease the divorce rate. I even talked a potential client out of divorce. Three times. Needless to say, I had to change careers.

Hey, if none of this works you can always move to a different country. I was five months pregnant when we first moved to Tanzania. It's not very common for foreigners to have their babies in country so I stood out like a sore thumb. In Tanzania, there are traffic police all over the place. They constantly pull you over to see if you have a proper driver's license and required fire hydrant. I've gotten to know a few of these officers quite well. We always enjoy a chat and they laugh at my pathetic attempts at Swahili.

A few months after I had the baby, I was pulled over by one of my favorite female police officers. I rolled down my window and she says, "I see you've remained fat!" Then gave me a huge high five. Voluptuousness is sacred here. I love it.

Group Discussion Questions:

1. How do you justify unhealthy choices in your head? What are your trigger statements?
2. It is ok to throw away food if it will cause you to overeat, even if you spent a lot of time or money on it. Discuss how you feel about this.
3. What are the parts of your body that you like? What type of exercise will help you punish the other parts to make them strong?
4. Why is confidence so important in your health journey?
5. How can y'all commit to helping each other realize your beauty and amazing capabilities?

CHAPTER THIRTY

YOU DESERVE CHOCOLATE

You deserve chocolate. You do! Honestly, you've had a stressful day, a stressful year, a stressful life! Chocolate will make you feel better. It absolutely will. Whoever said nothing tastes as good as thin feels is a dang liar. Sure, thin feels good. But holy Moses food tastes good.

You deserve chocolate for all the times you worked your butt off. You deserve chocolate for your "me time." You deserve chocolate for all the times you stopped at a stop sign! You deserve chocolate, darn-it. **But do you want it?**

Sure, a piece of chocolate every once in a while is not a big deal. Chocolate outside of moderation is a very big deal. Dessert is an acronym for: Death Encompassing Sweet Savory Everlasting Regrettable Torture. Say it three times fast. Truly, it is practically impossible to keep our calories under control with just our meals alone. So basically every time you have dessert you might be eating in a way that will cause you to gain weight. So how often do you have desserts, candy, sweets and the like?

If you continue to spike your insulin with processed sugars, it will hurt your body tremendously. Insulin affects so many processes in the body: hormones, mood, concentration, athletic ability, organ function, reproductive health, immune system, etc.

Foods that are acceptable in moderation are devastating in excess.

So let's get back to the chocolate. Take off two small squares, and put the rest of the bar in the freezer. I've found that if I keep the chocolate frozen, I'm not as tempted to get a piece. I've also found that if I eat dark chocolate, my chocolate craving is satisfied, and I'm not tempted to eat the entire chocolate bar in one sitting.

Lets say all of these precautions fail and you scarf down the entire bar of chocolate in five seconds flat. It happens. If it didn't, you wouldn't be reading this book. What should you do now? Set an alarm on your phone for one month and know that you are not allowed to have chocolate again until that month is over. Take all of the chocolate in your house and throw it away. Until you can refrain from overeating it, you shouldn't keep it around. Once you have healthy boundaries with chocolate, then you can easily put it back in your house. However, as long as it is causing you to destroy your physical and psychological health, don't burden yourself with the temptation.

Holidays are hard.

Holidays are notorious for inducing weight gain. Let's take a look at the major culprits: food, stress, and relationships.

Food. We live in a culture that celebrates everything with high calorie food, and lots of it. We live in a culture that has access to high calorie food at cheap prices and unnecessarily large portion sizes. The goal of holidays is to have the biggest, best, most savory dish that everyone will love. So food is part of the problem. Culture is part of the problem. Food culture is the problem.

Stress. There is so much pressure around Halloween, Thanksgiving, and Christmas. It's expensive: gifts, costumes, parties, travel, events, etc. It's busy: shopping, decorations, parties, church meetings, end of school semesters, traveling, cleaning your home for visitors, etc. It' extra: smelly candles, house decorations, car decorations, Christmas cards, traditions, holiday music, holiday food, holiday movies, work parties, family parties, friend parties, etc. It amazes me, but doesn't surprise me, that so many people feel depressed over the holidays.

Relationships. Say no more. Family obligations are thick. We are constantly aware of loved ones who are not around or those that were never there in the first place. We have to appropriately include everyone, because, Lord forbid, we hurt someone's feelings. We have to appropriately show our appreciation for everyone. All the times we have failed at relationships over the years are forever in your face. We are hurt when we aren't included, appreciated, or loved.

Here are a few quick tips to endure the holidays without putting on the holiday-hundred pounds.

1. It's ok to say no to food. Plan on turning down food. You will have to if you want to get through the holiday season in a healthy way. You can say

no to some things and enjoy others. Just don't eat everything that's offered.

2. It's ok to say no to people. Misery loves company. Emotional eaters don't like to eat alone. I'm guilty! But you don't have to hurt yourself to love others. Say no. Who knows, maybe you will inspire them to eat in moderation also.

3. Bring a healthy option. I love hummus and veggies. I always bring it to a party so I know I have something healthy to snack on for hours.

4. Eat before you go. Fill up on a protein and fibrous meal before you head out to the creamy creations of temptations. The less hungry you are, the better choices you will make.

5. Become a picky eater. Think about your absolute favorite holiday treat. Plan on having it. Then plan on saying no to everything else. Plan on how much you will eat and when you will eat it. Do not let anyone distract you from enjoying it. Savor every bite. Then, say no to everything else that is unhealthy.

6. Exercise. My favorite psychologist in the world Dr. Norman Lawson told me, "Walking eleven miles a week is as good for you as an anti-depressant." He meant me specifically, not someone who is clinically depressed and genuinely needs an antidepressant. Even still, clinically depressed friends can benefit from exercise. It reduces stress. It relaxes muscles. It releases happy endorphins. It burns extra calories (wink wink).

7. Brag about yourself. Tell everyone about your hard work. Seriously. Tell your co-workers, your

family, your friends, all the people you will be around, that you are trying to be more health conscious. Ask them to help you. Ask them to describe the food they are eating to you so you can enjoy it in your imagination while you are scarfing down carrot sticks. Ask them to sit with you somewhere that is not right by the Hanukkah cookies. You will be more likely to make healthy choices when you know people are on your side.

Once you make it through the holidays successfully, celebrate your self-control with two squares of that frozen chocolate.

Group Discussion Questions:

1. Have you ever had the courage to eat foods you absolutely love in healthy moderation? What strategies work for you?
2. Why are holidays difficult times to make healthy choices for you specifically?
3. What is your favorite holiday food?
4. What new traditions can you start that are not food-centric?
5. Do you want to be healthy more than you want to overeat?

CHAPTER THIRTY ONE

PUNCH SOMEONE

I'll tell you what, have you ever gone on a walk and the song Eye of the Tiger comes on? In that split second we all transform from a flabby middle-aged walker to a dynamite athlete. What is it about that song! One of my favorite things to do when I'm on stroll is to high-five people also out on an exercise stroll.

One day, it was beginning to get dark. I was strolling along a bayou trail near my house. I saw a little cute tween running towards me on the path. I was dressed in all black to help hide my sexy sweat stains. I got excited about my upcoming high five and picked up the pace. Eye of the tiger came on too. I was in the ZONE! As I approached this cute little jogger, I got closer to her side of the trail so we could make contact. At the last second I put up my hand and yelled, "Up top!"

Y'all, I have never seen a human jump so high. I scared the living daylights out of that girl! Poor thing. She took off running like the Flash! I'm pretty sure I yelled a little louder than I should have. I mean, Eye of the Tiger was playing y'all. If you happen to be reading this, pumpkin, I'm so sorry!

So what I'm saying is, punch people you run by. Wait, no, that is not what I'm saying. What I'm trying to say is:

To act differently you have to think differently.

In boxing, they say in order to defeat your opponent, destroy the head and the body will follow. Basically, if your opponent thinks they are weaker than you, then you will win. This is exactly how to address your health issues.

If you don't like where you're sitting, or the size of the booty you are sitting on, you need to start with the way you think. Defeat with you head. Get fed up with your opponent of oppressive thinking. Punch that burden right between the eyes. TKO baby!

What step do you need to take to think differently? What are you waiting for? A grim medical prognosis? I wish my dad hadn't waited that long. I miss him. Don't make the people you love miss you.

Get mad. Get tough. Get determined. Get angry! I'm angry that they've tripled the size of a fast food cheeseburger and soda in only twenty years. I'm angry my mom hated cooking and subconsciously made me dread cooking as an adult. I'm angry my natural eating habits keep me overweight, obsessed with food, and depressed.

I'm angry that I can be so fat and so hungry.

Does someone keep insulting you? Does someone laugh at you any time you talk about your health? Take those sad angry emotions and transfer that energy into productivity. Use it as fuel to do something about your health.

Are you stuck in a depression? Lack motivation? Go to a counselor and work on your mental health so you can take care of yourself. Don't have time to add anything "healthy" to your life? That's a lie. Watch a health documentary instead of playing on your phone. Change one meal a week to something healthy with protein, vitamins, and fiber. Pursue changing your mind so you can change your body. You can. You will.

And don't forget to high five a stranger. It is pretty fun.

Group Discussion Questions:

1. What is your favorite song to hear while you are exercising?
2. What beliefs hold you back from healthy choices?
3. What obstacles are you going to overcome to move toward the healthy life you truly long for?
4. What change can you make that will lead you down a healthier road?
5. Do you believe you can? Should you?

CHAPTER THIRTY TWO

FAST FOOD

I'll leave you with a few additional tips to encourage you on your health journey.

- Leave the last bite. Like pizza crust, for example. If you never ate pizza crust again you would save 52,000 calories a year. That's about fifteen pounds of fat EACH YEAR.
- Get an extra burger to go! And by that I mean, take half of your burger meal home. If you go out to a restaurant and order something unhealthy, then, when your meal arrives, immediately have the waitress put half the food in a to-go box. Drink a full cup of water before you eat from that box. I ordered a foot-long at Subway but the worker only gave me a six-inch. So she added a separate six-inch and they were wrapped separately. I guarantee you there is no way on God's green earth I was planning on eating only half of that sandwich. This time there was a natural pause after eating the first six-inch. I got distracted with something else. It just happened to be long enough for my body to realize I was actually full. I really enjoyed that free sandwich later and I enjoyed successfully cutting my meal calories in half.
- Cut Carbs. Ask yourself this question after every meal: How can I cut out carbs from this meal and still feel satisfied? You will find healthier alternatives that you don't mind. A few examples

include: spaghetti squash instead of noodles, cauliflower rice instead of regular rice, salad mix instead of tortillas.

- Make one small healthy change each day. If you are headed down a straight path, and you turn even a millimeter, you will eventually end up in a completely different place. If your current trajectory is unhealthy, just make a small change. A very small change can make a very big difference over time.

- Out of sight, out of mind. I asked my husband to freeze, hide, or throw away my trigger foods. If I leave chocolate on the shelf in the pantry, it will be the first thing I look for when I go into my pantry. So I either don't buy it at all, or I have my husband hide it so I have to ask him for it. I was considering investing in chocolate factories before I came up with this brilliant idea because of how much I consumed. Now, I hardly have it at all.

- Don't put it on the table. If you don't bring the pots of food to the table, then it won't be as easy to go back for seconds. You might actually find that you don't want them.

- Track your food and drink intake. Don't just write down what you eat; write down how you feel. It is important to keep a record of when unhealthy eating makes you feel terrible. Once you associate the food hangover with the food, you won't be as excited to scarf it down.

- Give up something. Maybe you can't give up sweets. Maybe you can't give up going back for seconds. That's fine! You can still find freedom in the way you eat. Give up the size of your plate then. Maybe if you eat dinner on a bread plate, then, when you get seconds; you are not overdoing your portion size times two and you're actually having a normal portion size. Maybe you cannot give up sweets but you can give up how often you eat them. Find something that you can give up that doesn't hurt to do. Once we get those knocked out, then we can work on the harder stuff.

- Stop eating when you stop tasting. This one is solid gold. If we are eating unhealthy foods because they taste good, then stop eating them when you stop tasting them. Really pay attention to this. That first cookie, so delicious. The second one? That processed food film starts to cover your taste buds. That third one? The taste isn't nearly as good. Stop eating. Then cleanse your palate with some refreshing fibrous food like cucumber, apple, carrots and the likes. Just don't go back to the cookies. Wait for another day.

- Get educated. Did you know what you eat affects all sorts of mood disorders? Depression, ADHD, anxiety, etc. Did you know cancer loves to feed off sugar? Did you know blueberries and spinach have antioxidants that repair some carcinogenic cells that would otherwise lead to cancer?

- Don't try to be someone else. Just try to be a better version of yourself. Comparison is just a big distraction. What health goals do you want for yourself? Stay focused on that and celebrate your achievements.

- You say you can't... Well, if someone was going to blow torch your eyes if you ever ate cake again, would you eat cake? Or if you would inherit a billion dollar trust fund if you got your BMI into the normal range, would you be able to then? You can. You can do hard things.
- Find your motivations and then put reminders everywhere. If it is your kids, put pictures of your kids on the fridge or in your car. If it's your medical diagnosis, put copies of it where your biggest temptations come from.
- Cut out one thing at a time. I ate a huge delicious brownie and still lost half a pound that week. How? Overtime I had eliminated foods that were high in carbohydrates that I didn't care for that much. I didn't eat toast that week. I had tacos on salad instead of in tortillas. So figure out what you can't live without, and live without the rest of the unnecessary calories.
- Stop drinking diet sodas. When your body thinks it's receiving glucose, and it doesn't, it then begins to crave sugar. I was having uncontrollable sugar cravings. A few weeks after I switched from diet sodas to plain soda water, I stopped having uncontrollable sugar cravings. No joke.
- Just because others are eating doesn't mean you have to eat. You might not believe me, but I promise you can sit through a meal where everyone has dessert and you decline. When I first took this kind of step in my health journey, it really helped to have SOMETHING even if it wasn't dessert. So I would get a cup of fruit or a

cup of coffee. Something that would keep my food cravings occupied to get me through the difficulty of skipping dessert.
- TASTE the foods you love. EAT the food that fuels you. Put one bite's worth of pie on your plate. Then fill up your plate with fruits, veggies, and proteins. You can still enjoy your favorite foods. Just don't make them the only foods you eat.

Forgiven and free.

F-words again. Forgive yourself for the harmful choices of the past. Be free to make better choices in the future. You won't be perfectly healthy every second for the rest of your life. It's OK! Just take a deep breath, and keep moving forward.

If you're not all in you don't have to be all out.

Maybe this season of life isn't the best to make a big transformation. That doesn't mean it can't be the season of life to make *some* healthy changes. You CAN enjoy eating healthy and exercising. I'm living proof. Take it one bite at a time. Go get 'em, tiger!

CHAPTER THIRTY THREE
OH LAWD!

Save the best for last right? As I write this last chapter, I'm sitting inside a McDonalds. The irony is not lost on me. Poor McDonalds. I feel like they only get bad press. They really are trying to make their menu healthier and I applaud them for that. [Pretend there is a really good transition sentence here to go into the next paragraph because, frankly, I just can't think of one.]

In the bible it says, "The fear of the Lord is the beginning of knowledge, but fools despise wisdom and instruction." Proverbs 1:7. The bible is full of wisdom about why we should take care of our bodies and how to do so.

I was already overweight the first time I read, the fruit of the Spirit is self-control. A very rough interpretation of this: if you believe in God then you will exhibit self-control. I had tons of it! In every area of my life except for eating: where I had none of it. It was tempting to believe that God wasn't real after all because I certainly didn't have what was promised. Instead, I believed it was true. That was the beginning of conviction: the beginning of freedom from gluttony. I realized something was wrong. I realized God wanted something better for me. I knew there was something more...

Think about fruit. How many things have to happen before a plant bears fruit? A seed must find it's way into the soil. It must get Son. Oops! I mean sun. It needs water. The seed eventually turns into a plant. That plant needs years of growth before it bears fruit. Finally the fruit comes.

Fruit itself is so beautiful. It sustains the lives of other creatures. It contains the seeds that are necessary to create new life. But before it can create new life, the fruit has to die. Then it's seeds will fall to the soil where the new life cycle begins.

Do you want the fruit of the Spirit of self-control? Do you want to have a healthy life-style and feel free? God wants that for you too.

After discovering this truth, I knew part of me had to "die." My expectation that I should just be healthy without trying had to die. My pride that I could do things on my own had to die. My denial that being overweight wasn't a big deal died a slow painful death.

What needs to die in your way of thinking?

The statement, "I just need more Jesus" is a false theology. If you are a believer in Jesus and you have walked from death to life, then you already have all of Jesus. If you are walking in sin in an area of your life, it is because you don't believe. It is not because you need "more" Jesus. So why don't you have more self control? What lies are you believing?

Here are some of the lies I believed that were preventing me from living in the fullness of the fruit of the Spirit of self control: God didn't have enough time for me. God was mad at me for my sin. God wouldn't heal me until I went to Heaven. God had more important things to do. Escaping with food would make me feel better. God wouldn't help me with my health because being overweight was keeping me humble. I was being punished for my sin and the sins of generations before me. All lies.

Jesus tells us He is "the way, the truth, and the life." Jesus says, "I've come so that you may have life and have it to the full." I wish he meant being full of cookie cake. He doesn't. That would actually be terrible for us. It is not our Heavenly Father's desire that we hate ourselves or that we live with the burden of being overweight. It is His desire to give us freedom. Regarding our health more specifically: freedom that comes only with self-control. Self-control is not a bad word. It is actually the road to freedom.

Once you find the source of your unbelief, then submit it to God. He is waiting for you; arms of love and healing open wide.

My children have such a hard time when I tell them no. They think my "no" means I don't love them. The opposite is true: because I love them, I say no. No, you cannot run out into a busy street. No, you can't jump off a 15-foot tree branch. No, you can't jump into the deep end of the pool until you know how to swim. You get the point.

No, you can't eat whatever you want, whenever you want, and stay healthy. Unless of course you eat like a rabbit, then by all means go ahead. But seriously, there is freedom in self-control. That is not how we see it though. We see it as restraint, punishment, even bondage. We see self-control the same way my kids saw my control.

Do you want life to the fullest?

In the health context, what does that mean? For me, it means enjoying food, having a healthy body, and not having feelings of guilt, shame or self-loathing around what I eat. It means healthy choices come naturally. I believe this is possible now, more than ever.

"If any of you lacks wisdom, you should ask God, who gives generously to all without finding fault, and it **WILL** be given to you." James 1:5 [emphasis added]. When was the last time you asked God for help? Sometimes I have to do it a hundred times a day.

If it really is true, that God created everything in the universe and every part of us (body, mind, soul), then doesn't it make sense that He cares about your health struggle? Doesn't an artist care if their art is being destroyed? If it really is true that God gave us words to learn about him and about life, don't you think he wrote a ton about how to take care of our bodies, the very vessel of the Holy Spirit? Would you tell someone to come visit you without giving them directions? If it really is true that Christ sets us free from Sin, then shouldn't He be the very first source that you seek to help you on your health journey?

He is the one that can set you free from vanity.

He can set you free from gluttony.

He can set you free from pain and suffering.

He can heal your mind.

He can heal your body.

If you believe in Him, He is already healing your soul.

Why are you running to so many other things instead of running straight into the arms of your Creator? Are you mad at me for making this accusation? Anger is a secondary emotion. If you feel angry, it's probably because there is truth somewhere in this accusation. Press in. What lies do you believe that are keeping you in the bondage of unhealthiness?

I truly believe without Jesus, I never would have been set free from the self-indulgent, emotional eating, over-weight hot mess that I was. But I do believe in Jesus. The only words to describe me now are Full & Free.

If you want to learn more about Jesus, I'd be happy to talk with you and get you pointed in the right direction to a good local church. Feel free to reach out to me on any social media platform. I can't wait to meet you.

HEY THANKS

First, thank you!

Thanks for hanging in there with me until the bitter end. Thank you for sharing your journey with me. Thank you for taking this time to care for yourself. Thanks for caring for yourself so you can better care for others.

If this book was the slightest bit helpful to you, would you consider buying it for someone else who is on a health journey? Sure, you could loan them your copy, but then you wouldn't have these tips to come back to whenever you needed a pick-me-up.

Also, I'll tell you exactly why you should buy this book again: so I can become a bagiliozilatatunionaire. Just kidding. I genuinely want to help the western world find their joy in being healthy. I want to save families from hundreds of thousands of dollars in medical bills because of bad habits. I want to bless grandchildren with the long lives of their healthy grandparents. I also want to provide for the third world. Is that term even politically correct? My time living in Africa has exposed me to some very painful truths about this world. I want to share the blessings I've been given to provide for those who are suffering more devastatingly than most of my readers can even imagine.

And I would really love to buy a fancy dog.

To my daddy, right before you passed away I asked you to ask Jesus to help me with my health. You must have. Thanks daddy. Thanks Jesus.

To my husband. You're hot. Thank you for loving Jesus. Thank you for all the hours we talked about this book. Thank you for supporting me every time you had to hide the cookies. Thank you for making me feel just as beautiful at 215lbs as 155lbs. Thanks for texting me on my long runs. Thanks for watching the kids while I exercised. Thanks for encouraging me to spend money on learning how to be healthier. Thank you for always being excited with me about whatever dream I was dreaming. Thank you for being proud of me. I can't wait to spend the rest of our lives together.

To my kids, may your days be full of properly portioned pieces of cake with giant satisfied smiles on your face.

To my mama, thanks for cooking for me every single day. Thanks for making veggies with every meal. Thanks for putting cheese on the broccoli. Thanks for being my #1 fan no matter what I do. I love you more than sky times earth.

To Amy Smith, my soul sister. Thanks for helping me to love salads. Thanks for always being my biggest fan. With you, it was never "if" I could and was always "when" I would.

To my editors, Lena Wensel and Jeanine Miller. I loved laughing with you, being criticized constructively by you, and just enjoying friendship with you. You are my faves. And thanks for helping me cuss a little less ;)

To hummus & carrots, thank you for saving me from hundreds of thousands of unwanted fat cells. You my BAE.

You can find more from Charlie Goodnight at:

charlie.goodnight.writer@gmail.com
facebook.com/AuthorCharlieGoodnight/
Twitter: @CharliGoodnight
Instagram: Charlie_goodnight